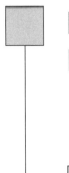

RESEARCHING
PALLIATIVE CARE

FACING DEATH

Series editor: David Clark, Professor of Medical Sociology, University of Sheffield

The subject of death in late modern culture has become a rich field of theoretical, clinical and policy interest. Widely regarded as a taboo until recent times, death now engages a growing interest among social scientists, practitioners and those responsible for the organization and delivery of human services. Indeed, how we die has become a powerful commentary on how we live and the specialized care of dying people holds an important place within modern health and social care.

This series captures such developments in a collection of volumes which has much to say about death, dying, end-of-life care and bereavement in contemporary society. Among the contributors are leading experts in death studies, from sociology, anthropology, social psychology, ethics, nursing, medicine and pastoral care. A particular feature of the series is its attention to the developing field of palliative care, viewed from the perspectives of practitioners, planners and policy analysts; here several authors adopt a multi-disciplinary approach, drawing on recent research, policy and organizational commentary, and reviews of evidence-based practice. Written in a clear, accessible style, the entire series will be essential reading for students of death, dying and bereavement and for anyone with an involvement in palliative care research, service delivery or policy making.

Current and forthcoming titles:

RESEARCHING PALLIATIVE CARE

Edited by
DAVID FIELD
DAVID CLARK
JESSICA CORNER
CAROL DAVIS

OPEN UNIVERSITY PRESS
Buckingham · Philadelphia

Open University Press
Celtic Court
22 Ballmoor
Buckingham
MK18 1XW

email: enquiries@openup.co.uk
world wide web: www.openup.co.uk

and
325 Chestnut Street
Philadelphia, PA 19106, USA

First Published 2001

A catalogue record of this book is available from the British Library

ISBN 0 335 20436 8 (pb)   0 335 20437 6 (hb)

Library of Congress Cataloging-in-Publication Data
Researching palliative care / edited by David Field . . . [*et al.*].
    p.   cm. – (Facing death)
    Includes bibliographical references and index.
    ISBN 0-335-20437-6 (hb) – ISBN 0-335-20436-8 (pbk.)
    1. Palliative treatment. 2. Terminal care. 3. Evidence-based medicine. I. Field, David, 1942– II. Series.
    R726.8.R465 2000
    362.1'75'072–dc21   00-044105

Typeset by Graphicraft Limited, Hong Kong
Printed in Great Britain by St Edmundsbury Press,
Bury St Edmunds, Suffolk

Contents

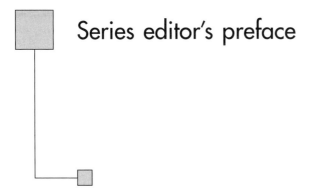

Series editor's preface

One particular concern of the Facing Death series is with the rapidly expanding field of palliative care. We began with an edited collection[1] which reviewed developments in the field from an international perspective. We followed this with a detailed sociological and policy analysis of palliative care in the UK context.[2] This new volume presented here, in which the editors draw attention to the specific field of palliative care research, complements the earlier two works admirably. It should be read by the growing number of academics, clinicians and planners who are concerned with the evidence underpinning palliative care, as well as that wider group of people who are interested in research relating to the field of death and dying more generally.

In the late 1950s and early 1960s the emerging territory of what was then called 'terminal care' first began to establish its claims to attention. One medium through which it did this was that of research. So it was that the work of early pioneers such as Cicely Saunders and John Hinton in Britain as well as Herman Feifel, Barney Glaser and Anselm Strauss in the United States came to be known and recognized.[3] From the outset however the significance of research was often overshadowed by more emotive appeals concerning the needs of dying people and those close to them. Indeed we might argue that the popular success of what came to be known as the hospice movement came about despite, rather than because of, the production of research based findings. Over time this position became less sustainable. In due course the recognition of palliative medicine as a specialty required that research finding, should be available to support both day to day clinical practice and wider service developments. More fundamentally still, in the 1990s, the culture of *evidence based healthcare* came into the ascendant and the impact of this on palliative care could not be avoided.

It was in the early 1990s that a nascent palliative care research community began to be recognizable. Academic departments of palliative care were formed, new journals appeared and there was increasing interest in the presentation of research findings at palliative care conferences. Interestingly, this community reflected some aspects of the wider culture of palliative care, in particular through its multi-disciplinary orientation. So it was sometimes possible to find physicians and nurses (though less frequently social workers and other professionals allied to medicine) working with social scientists in studies which addressed aspects of palliative care from a variety of perspectives. It was this willingness to work across disciplines which also facilitated a certain catholicity in the use of research methods. Nowadays multi-modal approaches are not uncommon in some areas of palliative care research and there are good examples of studies which have appropriately combined both qualitative and quantitative methods. In short, interest in palliative care research has never been stronger and that is why this new volume *Researching Palliative Care* has become necessary.

Who is the book intended to help?

It is no exaggeration to say that this book belongs on the shelves of anyone with an interest in the design, conduct and outcomes of palliative research. It has been edited by colleagues representing the disciplines of sociology, nursing and medicine. Together they have sought out a fascinating array of papers, all of them previously published, which when brought together in one volume, serve several purposes.

First, the book will help the novice researcher or even the person considering an initial foray into the world of palliative care research. It provides chapters on all the key research techniques which may be relevant, as well as some critical reflection on their robustness and applicability in particular contexts. It is not a handbook of research methods, but rather presents the reader with a stimulating range of possibilities along with illuminating editorial commentaries. Second, the book will I am sure be welcomed by those who are regularly engaged in and grappling with research problems in palliative care. It will provide a ready source of expert ideas and opinion on a range of commonly encountered research issues: from design, ethics approval, data collection, analysis and dissemination. Such readers will no doubt welcome the opportunity to have such a selection of key methodological papers in one convenient reference source. Third, the book will be extremely useful to those who teach on the growing number of masters courses in palliative care and related areas. Here is a core text for methods teaching which will aid both students and teachers alike. Finally, *Researching Palliative Care* will appeal to those practitioners, not necessarily involved in studies of their own, but who wish to better understand the veracity of evidence which is placed before them. These readers will find reassurance that the complexity of their clinical interventions is acknowledged by researchers who are in turn working hard to develop methodologies which are sufficiently sensitive to capture worthwhile findings.

The arrival of *Researching Palliative Care* within the Facing Death series is an important recognition of the role of research in this growing healthcare field. It marks a new maturity in palliative care research endeavours and at the same time points the way for further innovation and methodological refinement. It is a book of considerable practical relevance and also a challenging summation of the current state of the art. It demonstrates what palliative care research has achieved to date, but also underscores some of the problems and difficulties which have yet to be overcome.

David Clark

References

1 Clark, D., Hockley, J. and Ahmedzai, S. (1997) *New Themes in Palliative Care.* Buckingham: Open University Press.
2 Clark, D. and Seymour, J. (1999) *Reflections on Palliative Care: Sociological and policy perspectives.* Buckingham: Open University Press.
3 Clark, D. (1999) Cradled to the grave? Preconditions for the hospice movement in the UK, 1948–67. *Mortality,* 4(3): 225–47.

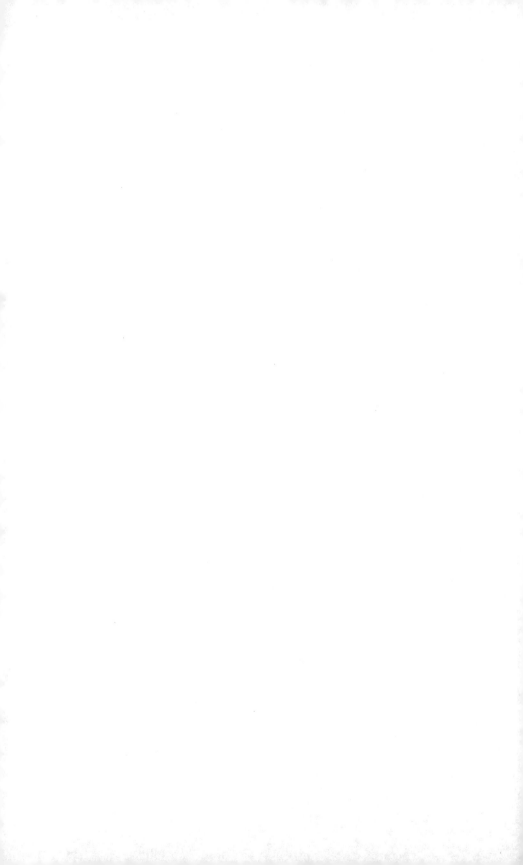

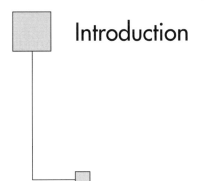

Introduction

The start of a new century prompts us to look ahead to future possibilities and to review our past. In palliative care there is a firm base of endeavour and achievement upon which to build and exciting possibilities for future development. The success of such developments will be influenced strongly by the excellence of the research base of palliative care. However, there are three main difficulties currently facing researchers in palliative care.[1] First, meeting the needs for care generally takes priority over establishing a sound research base for practice. While patient care will remain the priority, good quality research can contribute significantly to improving the quality of care and must be encouraged and supported. Second, research skills are lacking among palliative care professionals in all disciplines and at all levels, a difficulty this book aims to address. Third, palliative care settings tend to be relatively small and may be isolated from academic research institutions. During the 1990s, however, collaborative research between practitioners and researchers and between groups of researchers became more common, a few university-based research units dedicated to palliative care were established and such initiatives are likely to continue in the early decades of the new century. Other difficulties in conducting research in palliative care include the practical and ethical difficulties in studying those who are close to death, the lack of well-developed research instruments, and scarce research funding for palliative care. It is a sign of the increasing maturity of research in palliative care and the increasing importance given to such research that these difficulties have been identified and that ways to address them have become a subject for discussion at local and national levels.

This book is primarily intended as a resource for those directly involved in the delivery of palliative care who wish to pursue research but who have little or no formal training for or experience of conducting research. It is also intended as a resource for students on the increasing numbers of specialist palliative care courses, post-qualification short courses and taught Masters courses for health professionals which have 'health research skills' as important or central elements within their programmes. Although there are many general texts on research methods[2-6], there is only one methods text specifically addressing research issues in palliative care.[7] This book provides a resource for the improvement of research skills among researchers in palliative care by:

- identifying key issues in palliative care research;
- providing accessible examples and discussions of practical, methodological and ethical issues;
- presenting examples of good research practice;
- providing a wide-ranging coverage of the area;
- providing a resource for teachers and students.

Recognizing that palliative care research, training and practice often take place in institutions which do not have a substantial range of journals or basic research texts, this book covers the range of research methods that can appropriately be used for research in palliative care by reproducing previously published papers. This has the benefit of making these papers more easily accessible to a wide audience. We should note that we have chosen the papers to exemplify particular methods and topics which are central to research in the broadly conceived area of palliative care. They were selected on the basis of our collective knowledge of published research, consultation with colleagues who are experts in their areas of research, and after hand-searching key journals in palliative care. We identified many more suitable papers than we were able to accommodate, especially for Parts 2 and 3, and our choice was guided by consideration of the substantive focus and length of papers as well as by the chosen methods.

In this general introduction we will first discuss the development of research in palliative care and then consider some broad methodological considerations and approaches, relating these to issues for palliative care research. The introductions to the three sections of the book – key methods for researching palliative care; clinical research; needs assessment, audit and evaluation – will link these issues to the selected papers. The second and third sections also aim to cover a range of research topics within palliative care.

The development of research in palliative care

Research in palliative care can be traced back to the origins of palliative care in the modern hospice movement – conventionally defined as dating from the founding of St Christopher's Hospice in London in the 1960s.

From the very start, research was seen as one of the three 'legs' supporting hospice/palliative care (the others being holistic patient care and education).[8] Early research involved clinical studies of the effectiveness of treatment as well as narrative methods of talking to patients about their experiences of dying. The effective management of pain was a major focus of this research. As Corner[9] notes, these early studies were pivotal in establishing the speciality and provided powerful data about the needs of dying people. However, much of the research in palliative care has remained small scale and locally based and may be concerned mainly to identify local problems, with insufficient attention to how these might be dealt with at a national level. Despite the rapid growth in the number and range of palliative care services, and in the management and care of dying patients, rigorous evaluation of these developments or well-designed intervention studies have been most noticeable by their absence.

During the 1990s the demand for research in health care in the UK has been strengthened by health service reforms and driven by nationally set priorities focusing upon cost containment, evidence-based delivery of care and clear indicators of the outcomes and effectiveness of services.[10] Palliative care has not been immune to the demands of audit and research, especially as palliative care services in the voluntary sector are now part of the wider framework of health care commissioning and there has been a concomitant interest in strengthening the evidence-base. Higginson[11] has noted some difficulties in applying an evidence approach to palliative care. First, an absence of evidence does not mean that a service or treatment is ineffective and palliative care does appear to contain certain elements which are inherently difficult to measure. Second, significant problems have occurred when the 'gold standard' of the randomized controlled trial has been applied to palliative care services. Third, there are problems in measuring the quality of life of patients with progressive illness. These issues are addressed by some of the chapters in this book. Overcoming them will be an important prerequisite for the establishment of evidence-based palliative care.

Running alongside these developments within health services in Britain, palliative care has become increasingly formalized with a number of professional associations and interest groups emerging which, separately and working together, promote the speciality at local, regional and national levels. Interest in research is also increasing, indicated by the establishment of the Palliative Care Research Forum of Britain and Ireland in 1991 and the growth in attendance at its annual conferences and in its membership. Similarly, in 1996 the Association of Palliative Medicine formed a Science Committee and in 1997 the Royal Society of Medicine created a Palliative Care Forum. These developments and an emerging sense of collective identity have led to attempts to define the scope of research in palliative care. Thus, Corner[12] suggests palliative care research encompasses 'the total care of the patient whose disease is no longer responsive to curative treatment;

argued that there are potentially endless ways of knowing, understanding, experiencing and using physical phenomena and objects. Reality is *contingent* rather than *given*, and its effects and meanings for human behaviour depend upon the interactions between humans and their environment. These interactions are crucially shaped and directed by the use of language. In this view, reality is seen as *socially constructed* and variable. Within palliative care research (and within health services research more generally) this position is best represented by what is broadly categorized as 'interpretivist' or 'qualitative' research.[17] This approach emphasizes the importance of taking proper account of the ways in which research subjects make sense of their experiences. While positivist research aims to 'distance' the researcher from the collection of data by striving to maintain objectivity and 'value freedom', interpretivist research acknowledges that the interaction between those being researched and the researcher will affect what is found, and encourages 'self-reflexivity' as a way of incorporating and accounting for the subjective experiences of researchers into the research process and findings.

The main aim of qualitative research is to identify and explain underlying social processes and values, to link these to their social context and to develop higher level analytic categories from what is found. It aims to go beyond the 'surface' and easily observable aspects of reality to the 'private' experiences and meanings of individuals. The interaction between data collection and analysis is central to the research process and the qualitative researcher needs to be open to the unexpected. An important aspect of qualitative research is that it may be redirected through the process of research rather than, as in quantitative research, staying rigidly to its original focus and direction. Qualitative research involves personal involvement, and close relationships may develop between the researcher and the researched, which may generate ethical and personal difficulties.

This approach to the nature of reality and the role of research leads to a different attitude towards the issues of validity and reliability from that found within positivist research.[18] Qualitative researchers are concerned to capture what is going on accurately, but question the possibility of doing this through the procedures followed by quantitative researchers. Rather than refer to 'validity', it might be better to describe the goal of qualitative research as to provide coherent and adequate plausible explanations of human behaviour based on rigorous procedures of data collection and analysis. One way of tackling this is by reflecting explanations and findings back to the subjects of the research in order to assess whether they are accepted as recognizable and adequate. Reliability, as defined by positivists, is simply not a relevant concern for this type of research, focusing as it does upon the role of the researcher(s) in eliciting unique and variable meanings. The possibility of generalizing to other groups and settings is largely addressed by searching for common patterns across different research studies. Although there appears to be much greater diversity within qualitative research about how to judge the adequacy of its research, general rules have been developed to enable such evaluation.[19] As with quantitative research these focus largely upon the transparency of research methods and procedures and the integrity of researchers in their presentation and analysis of their findings.

These different approaches to understanding reality are reflected by different types of research topics and methods. The most obvious difference between qualitative and quantitative research is that the former concentrates upon people and their experiences and that it uses words rather than numbers as its data. Positivist or quantitative research studies are usually aimed at identifying or examining causal relationships between variables and attempt to analyse the probability or certainty of particular outcomes or relationships between variables through statistical analysis. They are deductive, framing their questions and hypotheses in terms of existing theory and knowledge. Typical research methods are randomized controlled trials, experiments and surveys based upon representative samples of a population. Interpretivist or qualitative research studies are concerned to study human experiences and subjective meanings and to locate these within their social context. Rather than testing theories and hypotheses they are inductive and concerned to discover new knowledge and to 'ground' this in the subjective experiences of their subjects. Typical research methods are participant observation, open-ended in-depth interviews, focus groups and case studies.

While it is useful to understand the underlying theories of knowledge which inform 'quantitative' and 'qualitative' research and how these affect research topics and methods, a rigid distinction between them is not helpful.[20] There are a variety of methods grouped under these broad categories and there are sometimes substantial differences between methods within each category. It is now widely accepted that quantitative and qualitative methods may be complementary and that it may be an advantage to combine them. This is sometimes referred to as 'method triangulation', where different methods are used to collect information about a topic. For example, a comparative study of the care of dying patients in their own homes and in a hospice might use well-validated clinical tests to gather 'objective' data about symptom management, standardized psychological scales to measure mental states such as anxiety and depression, a structured questionnaire administered to both groups of patients to gather information about the provision of services and in-depth open-ended interviewing of purposefully selected samples of patients and their relatives to collect information about their experiences of and satisfaction with care. Although some consideration needs to be given to the differences between approaches, there are no 'best' or 'worst' methods and in practice researchers are unlikely to decide upon their philosophical principles and then base their selection of research topic and methods upon these.

In palliative care, research topics are often practice-based and usually problem-led. Methods must be selected in light of the research problem, the speed with which results are wanted, the use to which they will be put, and the resources available. Sometimes, as suggested above, a combination of methods is the best research option. All research methods have their strengths and weaknesses, and it is impossible for the researcher to choose a method that is entirely without drawbacks or problems. While methodological considerations may steer the researcher towards one method or set of related methods rather than another, in choosing a method or methods the researcher must weigh the relative advantages and disadvantages of those that are available and choose those that are best for the research in question.

Selecting the appropriate research methods is not simply a matter of selecting the best methods to use on purely methodological grounds. There will also be a number of sometimes obdurate and/or conflicting practical considerations, which must be addressed. Put simply, these concern the nature and amount of resources available and gaining access to research subjects and relevant information. It is a very rare research project which has no time, labour or technical support constraints, and research in health care is likely to encounter ethical dilemmas which may only be resolved in ways which place constraints upon the methods which can be used. Thus, the choice of research methods will be constrained by the time which is available for the research; the number and skills of the researchers; the nature and extent of secretarial, computing, statistical and transcription support; restrictions which may be placed upon access to research subjects and to written and statistical information. Access to potential subjects and information may also be constrained by the amount of travelling required to conduct interviews and to visit research sites. There may also be conceptual difficulties in defining key concepts (e.g. 'satisfaction' or 'quality of life') and in establishing appropriate measurable outcomes. These conceptual difficulties are more likely to be found in new and developing areas of research, such as in palliative care.

There are a number of common problems that it is particularly important for researchers in palliative care to consider. Many of these concern the difficulties of gaining information directly from people who are dying. The ethical and practical difficulties of research involving patients who are close to death should not be underestimated. There may be ambivalence from care staff about asking their patients to participate in studies requiring time, effort and sometimes discomfort. The instability of their disease condition in a high proportion of eligible patients may confound the ability to assess the effect of the treatment(s) or intervention(s) being studied and may also make it difficult to achieve sufficiently high sample sizes to allow statistically significant results to be reported. It may also be difficult to follow up patients over a sufficiently long period of time and attrition of patients as a result of death or deterioration in health during the study may be high. Thus, samples are likely to be atypical of the population of patients receiving palliative care. For these reasons, many researchers use relatives and/or other carers to report on patients' experiences, opinions and attitudes towards their care.

We can identify the main problems for research in palliative care as:

- attrition of subjects through illness progression and death;
- ethical issues of involving dying and bereaved people in research, especially when there is no immediate benefit to them from the research;
- the role of 'gatekeepers' (especially doctors and nurses) who mediate/enable access to patients and their 'lay carers';
- the use of surrogate accounts for patient experiences and opinions;
- definition of key concepts (e.g. quality of life, palliative care, terminal care);
- selecting appropriate measures;
- establishing appropriate outcomes for evaluating palliative care.

Summary

There is a range of methods that can be used for researching palliative care. Good research will match methods to the aims and purpose of the research project. It will be clear, rigorous and open in its description of its methods; clear and honest in its presentation of findings; and self-reflexive and critical in its discussion of the implications and wider generalizabilty of those findings. All methods and research tools have their weaknesses as well as their strengths but research methods themselves are neither intrinsically 'right' nor 'wrong'. There may be good and bad *use* of methods and it is useful to understand the basic 'rules' which can be applied when implementing or evaluating any research. We have framed these as a set of questions:

- Is there an appropriate fit between the aims/purpose of the research and the method(s) used?
- Are the methods and their application described fully and clearly? Can the reader see what was done, how it was done and why it was done in this way?
- Is the research rigorous and systematic? Are the 'rules' for the research explained clearly and defensibly?
- Is the research ethically sound?
- Is there openness and transparency in the reporting of the analytic procedures used and the presentation of results?
- Can the reader make an informed assessment of the adequacy of the research methods and procedures?

- Are the results presented clearly and appropriately?
- Are the interpretation and discussion of findings consistent with the methods adopted and the evidence presented?

References

1   Richards, M.A., Corner, J. and Clark, D. (1998) Developing a research culture for palliative care. *Palliative Medicine*, 12: 399–403.
2   Bickam, L. and Rog, D.J. (eds) (1998) *Handbook of Applied Social Research Methods*. London: Sage.
3   Bowling, A. (1997) *Research Methods in Health: Investigating Health and Health Services*. Buckingham: Open University Press.
4   Daly, J., McDonald, I. and Willis, E. (eds) (1992) *Researching Health Care: Designs, Dilemmas and Disciplines*. London: Tavistock/Routledge.
5   Denscombe, M. (1998) *The Good Research Guide*. Buckingham: Open University Press.
6   Seale, C. (ed.) (1998) *Researching Society and Culture*. London: Sage.
7   Robbins, M. (1998) *Evaluating Palliative Care: Establishing the Evidence Base*. Oxford: Oxford Medical Publications.
8   Clark, D. and Seymour, J. (1999) *Reflections on Palliative Care: Sociological and Policy Perspectives*. Buckingham: Open University Press.
9   Corner, J. (1996) Is there a research paradigm for palliative care? *Palliative Medicine*, 10: 201–8.
10 Clark, D. and Seymour, J. (1999) Op. cit.
11 Higginson, I. (1999) Evidence based palliative care. *British Journal of Medicine*, 319: 462–3.
12 Corner, J. (1996) Op. cit.
13 Hughes, J. (1990) *The Philosophy of Social Research*, 2nd ed. London: Longman.
14 Seale, C. (ed.) (1998) Op. cit.
15 Seale, C. (1999) *The Quality of Qualitative Research*. London: Sage.
16 Seale, C. (1998) Op. cit.
17 Mays, N. and Pope, C. (eds) (1996) *Qualitative Research in Health Care*. London: BMJ Publishing Group.
18 Seale, C. (1999) Op. cit.
19 Ibid.
20 Bryman, A. (1998) *Quantity and Quality in Social Research*. London: Unwin Hyman.

PART I

Key methods for researching palliative care

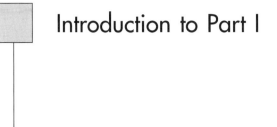

Introduction to Part I

The chapters in this opening section of the book provide an introduction to the main research methods which are used in researching different aspects of palliative care. Although it is not a comprehensive coverage, our selection is intended to present the reader with clear examples of key methods, their strengths and weaknesses, and how they may be used. The chapters in the subsequent sections of the book use many of the methods described here.

It is useful to conduct a thorough review of the relevant literature prior to beginning research. The systematic review takes this initial step of reviewing literature to its most developed form. In the opening selection Hearn, Feuer, Higginson and Sheldon provide a clear account of how to conduct a systematic literature review as well as providing a useful set of references for further help and information. Systematic reviews aim to identify, evaluate and synthesize research evidence in order to provide empirical answers to research questions. They can thus be a useful tool to provide access to potentially unmanageable amounts of research evidence. Central features of a systematic review are the clear and precise definition of the research question, the identification of all relevant sources of literature and the systematic and thorough electronic and hand searching of this literature. In a systematic review the usual partial and potentially slanted selection of papers is replaced by a comprehensive review of the literature within the relevant area which applies clear criteria for the selection of studies and for their discussion in a systematic manner. With the apparently exponential expansion of research evidence in palliative care, the systematic review has become recognized as an important way for researchers and practitioners to keep abreast of new developments. The chapter by Hearn and Higginson in Part II provides a good example of a systematic review.

One commonly used method of gathering information about the experience of receiving palliative care services is the social survey. The main instrument for collecting information in the social survey is a schedule of questions, although other instruments such as Likert scales and visual analogues may also be used. Developing appropriate, valid and reliable questions is a skilled task, so first-time and novice researchers will often use questionnaires developed for other research studies either directly, or modified to take account of their particular context and research aims. Surveys may make use of three possible approaches: face-to-face interviewing; self-completion of a postal questionnaire; or telephone interviews. In social surveys, interviews are usually based on a structured schedule of 'closed format' questions that can be pre-coded to allow for data entry and computer analysis. Some face-to-face surveys of sensitive topics are now making use of technologies which allow respondents to enter their responses directly on to a laptop computer, thus preserving the confidentiality of their responses. The schedule may also contain some 'open-ended' questions to allow respondents to expand upon their answers and to express their own views and experiences. Closed-format questions depend to a large extent on prior knowledge and information about what is to be studied (although not necessarily in a detailed way). When little is known about the research area non-directive, qualitative, interviews using 'open-ended' questions may be a better technique for gaining an understanding of attitudes and beliefs, and how these influence and are influenced by experiences and behaviour. This method is also suitable for use when researching sensitive, stigmatized, intensely personal, or potentially embarrassing subjects. Put simply, structured interviews focus on known possibilities and lines of action while unstructured interviews are likely to be used when the researcher does not know the answer and/or wants to discover people's own meanings and interpretations. We do not include a selection on interviewing, but these are well summarized in Denscombe's *Good Research Guide*.[1]

Given the many practical difficulties and ethical concerns about approaching dying people directly for their views, surveys of palliative care frequently use their relatives to provide information. Some of the most important research evidence we have in the UK about terminal care comes from social surveys using this approach.[2] This is not without its problems, and in the second chapter in this section Addington-Hall and McCarthy draw upon the largest UK national survey study using this approach to provide a clear account of the rationale and issues to be addressed in interview-based survey research with bereaved relatives. Hinton examines the validity of using relatives to 'speak' for dying people in the second section of this book. Useful evidence on palliative care services can be collected by small-scale, locally based surveys, as Addington-Hall and McCarthy argue. The utility of such surveys depends crucially upon selecting the right sample and one question that is frequently asked is, 'How many subjects are needed in a research sample?' This is discussed by Faithfull in the subsequent chapter.

Within medicine, the use of placebos in randomized 'double-blind' clinical trials (i.e. where nobody knows whether the drug or a placebo is being administered) is generally regarded as the 'gold standard' for clinical research. Within palliative care, there is no such consensus. We first examine the issues of placebo-controlled trials in palliative care by presenting in this section the arguments 'for' and 'against' their use. Hardy presents the case 'for', arguing they offer the greatest scientific rigour and will thus provide a strong evidence base for palliative care. She acknowledges the practical difficulty of recruiting sufficient numbers of palliative care patients to make this viable, and Part II includes an account of her difficulties in using this research design. In response to Hardy, Kirkham and Abel identify a number of problems in conducting placebo-controlled trials in palliative care and also point to some technical issues which make it difficult to rely upon such trials to provide good evidence to inform palliative care practice. They argue that there are other ways of assessing how well a drug works with palliative care patients.

Most health services research, including that in palliative care, is based on the use of quantitative methods such as those reviewed above. However, within palliative care qualitative research has always played an important role. Perhaps the best known and most widely cited qualitative study is that by the US sociologists Glaser and Strauss[3] which identified the central importance of communication and awareness of dying for cancer patients. The methods they used in this study are the basis for 'grounded theory' – one of the most widely cited and commonly used approaches within qualitative research.[4,5] In his chapter Clark provides a brief background to the development of qualitative research in palliative care and discusses the techniques that make up the 'toolkit' of qualitative research – observation, participant observation, qualitative interviews, focus groups, documentary analysis and case studies. Clark argues that there is a set of recognizable and rigorous procedures which are followed in good qualitative research and that such research has great potential for further development in palliative care.

Research involving palliative care patients inevitably raises ethical issues, some of which are referred to in a number of the chapters in this book. This section therefore closes with a chapter by Wilkie, the Chair of a local Research Ethics Committee, who summarizes the key ethical issues which researchers in palliative care must address in their research in a clear and useful manner. Although her focus is qualitative research, the general principles of balancing benefits and risk, the issues of patient consent and participation, deception, confidentiality and the effect of the research upon the patients also apply to quantitative research. For example, 'Phase 1' research trials into the relative effectiveness of different drugs or treatment regimes when no clinical benefit can be guaranteed for the patient must clearly address these issues.

Although we have been unable to cover all of the research methods which could be used in palliative care research, the chapters in this section provide a good introduction to the most commonly used methods. The chapters in the next two sections provide further examples of these and demonstrate their application to specific areas within palliative care. If, as we hope, palliative care is to continue its growth and development, soundly based research of current and emerging issues will be essential to inform practice and policy.

References

1 Denscombe, M. (1998) *The Good Research Guide*. Buckingham: Open University Press.
2 Seale, C. and Cartwright, A. (1994) *The Year Before Death*. Aldershot: Avebury.
3 Glaser, B.G. and Strauss, A.L. (1965) *Awareness of Dying*. Chicago, IL: Aldine.
4 Denscombe, M. (1998) Op. cit.
5 Seale, C. (1999) *The Quality of Qualitative Research*. London: Sage.

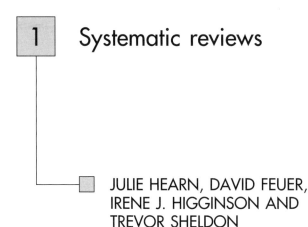

1 Systematic reviews

JULIE HEARN, DAVID FEUER,
IRENE J. HIGGINSON AND
TREVOR SHELDON

The volume of biomedical literature published annually is currently increasing at an exponential rate. Over two million articles in 20,000 journals are published annually.

The traditional way for doctors and nurses to keep in touch with this expansive literature has been a 'narrative' review, editorial, or book chapter, in which an expert in the field is asked for his or her expert opinion. The problems with this approach are now clear. This type of review is subjective and prone to severe bias and error.[1] Selective inclusion of studies that support the author's view is common – the frequency of citation of clinical trials is related to their outcome, with studies in line with the prevailing opinion being quoted more frequently than unsupportive studies.[2] Equally, opposite conclusions are often reached[3] with reviews by different authors in different journals without it being clear why, and some of the small yet potentially important differences are often missed.[4] In controversial areas where practice differs, the conclusions drawn from a given body of evidence may be associated more with the speciality of the reviewer than with the available data.[5] Within palliative medicine, different reviews have suggested both the efficacy or not of transcutaneous electrical nerve stimulation in chronic pain,[6,7] and the efficacy or not of treating recurrent malignant bowel obstruction with surgery.[8,9] 'Expert opinion' often lags behind the research evidence and is not infrequently inconsistent with it.

Systematic reviews aim to locate, appraise and synthesize research evidence from scientific studies to provide informative empirical answers to scientific

---

Box 1.1   Advantages of a systematic review

- Unmanageable quantities of research on a topic are found, summarized, appraised and communicated to decision makers, researchers and health care providers.
- 'New' information is provided (by increasing power and precision), which may not be apparent from individual studies where effects and investigation are small. The consequent delays in implementation of the results may therefore be reduced.
- Explicit methods limit bias and errors, limiting prejudice, unconscious bias, incomplete knowledge and appropriate weighting of data.
- The conclusions and reproducibility of the results are reliable and accurate.
- The results of different studies can be formally compared to establish generalizability of findings and consistency of results (homogeneity).
- Reasons for heterogeneity (differences in results across studies) can be identified and new hypotheses generated.

---

research questions.[10,11] Therefore, they are a scientific tool which can be used to summarize the results and implications of otherwise unmanageable quantities of research. They differ from earlier types of review in that they adhere to a strict scientific design in order to make them more comprehensive, to minimize the chance of bias, and so ensure their reliability. Rather than reflecting the prior views of the authors or being based on a biased selection of the published literature, each systematic review follows a protocol with clearly defined questions and explicit methodology, thereby providing a comprehensive summary of the available evidence.[12,13] In addition to providing a better basis for clinical practice, systematic reviews also identify gaps in the research, enabling future research priorities to be set in an objective way. The advantages of systematic reviews are listed in Box 1.1.

The characteristics of the systematic review are:

- clearly stated questions and objectives;
- a comprehensive strategy to search the literature for studies that address the objectives of the review, to include unpublished as well as published studies;
- explicit and justified criteria for the inclusion or exclusion of any studies;
- a comprehensive list of all studies identified;
- clear presentation of the characteristics of the studies included, and an analysis of methodological quality;
- a comprehensive list of all studies excluded, and justification for exclusion;

- clear analysis of the results of eligible studies, with statistical synthesis of data (meta-analysis if appropriate and possible);
- sensitivity analysis of the synthesized data if appropriate and possible;
- structured report of the review, clearly stating the aims, describing the methods and materials, and reporting the results.

Systematic reviews should be reliable summaries of research evidence. They are particularly useful when there is uncertainty regarding the potential benefits or harm of an intervention, when there are variations in practice, and when research is being planned. They are a basis for informing best practice.[14–16] This chapter illustrates the role of conducting systematic reviews in the area of palliative care.

Defining the question

The question is normally stated in terms of:

- the patient or population;
- the intervention or exposure that is being analysed;
- the clinical outcome.

It is these three areas together with methodological criteria that become the inclusion criteria for the review. In a recent systematic review, 'The effects of fluid status and fluid therapy on the dying', the population was terminally ill patients, the intervention was fluid therapy and outcomes were those reported in the studies, e.g. symptom distress.[17]

The topic to be reviewed can be further divided into discrete research questions. This is termed 'operationalizing the review'. For example, if we were to conduct a review of pain control in palliative care the focus of the review may be on the effectiveness of a health technology, such as syringe drivers for pain control, or on different strategies to combat the problem, such as using drug versus behavioural therapies for pain control, or to answer questions regarding the organization of health care, for example, comparing team working versus specialized individuals' effectiveness at controlling pain.

One area reviewed as part of producing national guidance on commissioning colorectal and lung cancer services in England[18–21] was communication, an issue which relates to the organization of health care. Poor communication with cancer patients is one of the most common causes for litigation or complaint.[22] The hypothesis that there are problems related to communication with patients with cancer and their families was subdivided into two sections and operationalized into the questions given in Box 1.2.

Box 1.2   Operational interpretation of the proposal to review communication

(1) *Is there a problem?*
  • Do patients with lung cancer and their families/carers experience suboptimal communication?
  • Is there a lack of communication between professionals, both within and between settings?
  • What methods of information giving exist to improve communication; how effective are they?
  • What effect does poor communication have on the health of the patient and family?
  • Do specialist nurses improve the flow of information?
(2) *What training is there; does it work?*
  • What methods have been proposed for education and training of health care professionals in information giving to patients with cancer?
  • Is there any evidence that training increases the ability of health care professionals to give information?

Searching the literature

Once the questions have been determined and a protocol devised following guidance laid out in reports such as those produced by the NHS Centre for Reviews and Dissemination,[23] or the Cochrane Collaboration,[24] the search for research evidence begins. The aim of searching is to provide as comprehensive a list as possible of relevant primary studies, both published and unpublished, which may fit the inclusion criteria for the review. The precision of the final estimate of effectiveness will depend on the volume of information obtained, hence it is important that the search for primary studies is extensive.[25]

Electronic databases

Major electronic databases [MEDLINE, EMBASE, the Cochrane Library, the Database of Abstracts of Reviews of Effectiveness, and Nursing and Allied Health (CINAHL)], do not cover the same source material or have the same indexing. Therefore, for a comprehensive search more than one database should be accessed.[26] There are also many specialist databases, such as CANCERLIT, PSYCHLIT, AIDSLINE and AGELINE, each with their own idiosyncrasies. It is essential to involve specialist librarians in the search process, as they are trained to search efficiently, and have a wide knowledge of information resources. Librarians need to be budgeted for in the project protocol.

The keywords of seminal papers in the field are a useful starting point for constructing a search strategy. However, searching on textwords can improve the sensitivity of searches given the variable indexing of papers.[27] Searching databases can be very time-consuming, particularly if computer software crashes. It is helpful to record search strategies, both as a method of recording progress, and to enable searches to be repeated with ease. The problem with electronic searches is that a high recall strategy implies low precision, and equally a high precision search will result in low recall. A balance needs to be struck to ensure that the search is relatively comprehensive, but that there are not unmanageable amounts of inappropriate references.

The failure of electronic databases to find all the relevant studies on one topic was illustrated in the systematic review on methodological issues in effectiveness research on palliative cancer care. Searching all the major computer databases from 1966 to 1985 only revealed half of the 11 studies the authors eventually extracted from the literature.[28] Unfortunately, papers are often poorly indexed by journals, and some journals are not yet on electronic databases. Clearly other sources of information may need to be searched in order that the evidence presented is as complete as possible, including the handsearching of high-yield journals.

Handsearching

Although electronic databases provide a relatively simple and quick method of searching for papers, handsearching journals can often provide you with additional studies missed during database searching, or containing data on the topic of interest within a study that had a different focus.

Based on the number of relevant studies identified through other means, and considering resources available, a decision must be made as to which journals and how many years will be searched as this can be a time-consuming process. Only those journals with a potentially high yield, for example specialist journals, should be searched.

Other sources

Consultation with other experts in the field can yield as yet unpublished data, or grey literature, such as reports, dissertations or theses. The SIGLE database may provide an easier route for finding grey literature. Scanning reference lists can be useful for locating studies in newer journals which may not be included on some databases. Conference abstracts can be useful for identifying the most up-to-date research, which may since have been published.

Loitering in libraries

The next stage of a review involves retrieving the papers. With the increase in the number of online journals, including the *British Medical Journal*,[29] and the *Journal of Public Health Medicine*,[30] getting full copies of recent articles is becoming easier. However, finding papers not online can be time-consuming. Not only do you need to locate a library that stocks the desired journal and which holds the relevant editions, an archived edition may need to be ordered from the librarian (which can take up to several hours), or the required edition may be being bound/not on the shelf/being used by someone else. Alternatively, interlibrary loans can be ordered, but these are time-consuming and expensive.

Do not underestimate the time that will be spent both travelling between libraries, and loitering in them. Interlibrary loans and other document retrieval services provided by libraries can be used to overcome these issues, but can be expensive and should be accounted for in the budget for the review.

During the search for research evidence there will be a continuous trade-off between validity versus workload, and decisions need to be made between time or resources and comprehensiveness. At whatever point searching is stopped, it is important to be explicit about the methods used when reporting the review to enable it to be repeated and thereby updated.

Inclusion/exclusion

It is important to assess first the relevance of studies, to sort through and identify those which report evaluation that helps to answer one or more of the review questions, and exclude those of interest but which are truly not relevant. Clear criteria for relevance should be included in the protocol, and may include factors such as study design, participants, length of follow-up and the outcome measures used. This will result in a comprehensive list of studies.

Data extraction software such as RevMan[31] can be useful to ensure that all the research data are stored in a standardized way and can be analysed easily. However, other software, or tables in a word-processing package can be simple and efficient to use. Clarity and brevity are important at this stage – pose the question: 'Do I really want to rewrite every paper?' Provide sufficient detail to enable you to describe accurately and assess the results reported. An alternative to extracting into tables would be to use a comprehensive data extraction sheet to record information on a study, followed by summarizing this into a table. Whether this is appropriate or not is dependent on the type of data and number of studies being reviewed. It is important to bear in mind that the effectiveness of a health care intervention is likely to depend on 'a large number of factors relating to who receives it, who delivers it and how, and in what context'.[32]

Methodological quality

Many criteria exist to evaluate the quality of a study. It is this quality which allows us to gauge the likelihood of the results being a valid estimate of the truth, i.e. high-quality studies are said to give a more realistic estimate of treatment effects, are more accurate and reproducible, and there is therefore greater acceptance of their results by the medical and nursing establishment. For example, 25 scales and nine checklists exist to assess the quality of randomized controlled trials,[33] and apart from empirical evidence suggesting that allocation concealment and double blinding are associated with bias,[34] the other items on these checklists have little or no evidence to support their use. There is no validated 'gold standard' for the true methodological quality of a study.[35] Hence methodological hierarchies should not be applied slavishly. Ultimately, the aim is to identify those studies which, by virtue of their design and quality of conduct, analysis and reporting are the least biased and most reliable. This may vary according to what is being evaluated and the questions being asked.

Ideally, the decision to include studies and the extraction of data should be checked by using two reviewers, or having a random sample selected for reviewing a second time by someone else.

Carrying out systematic reviews in areas where more qualitative research has been conducted is quite difficult since criteria for appraising qualitative studies are still being developed, and qualitative studies are often prone to a poor quality of reporting.

Data synthesis

A qualitative analysis of the evidence is an essential step in the assessment of effectiveness of a health technology, and it is within this context that any quantitative synthesis should take place.

A qualitative overview considers all the results taking into account not only the methodological rigour, and therefore reliability of these studies, but also helping to highlight and explore differences.

The lack of randomized controlled trials in palliative care makes this process even more important. Stating how much information has been found and the grade of the evidence enables findings to be summarized in cases where meta-analyses or number needed to treat analyses cannot be performed.

Sensitivity analysis is the way in which different inclusion criteria, methods or assumptions can be analysed to see what effect they have on the results. An analysis may be carried out using all the studies found, and then again after removing certain studies. Examples include removing poorer quality studies, or by calculating the final effect size by a different statistical method, or using only the more recent published data or studies of a certain size. The final conclusion can be analysed to see if these variables will affect the result. If the overall result remains unchanged, one can conclude the results are relatively robust with regard to the various factors analysed. Equally, if the results are dramatically changed, i.e. by using smaller or the lower quality studies a profound and large effect compared to the larger or higher quality trials is seen, then these are sources of heterogeneity. They need to be investigated further, and the key findings of the review may need to be assessed more cautiously.

A Pain, Palliative Care and Supportive Care Collaborative Review Group has recently registered as part of the Cochrane Collaboration. This group aims to produce and maintain reviews in these areas, with the fundamental aim of benefiting patients who will 'have access to better evidence and receive treatment of proven benefit'.[36] To date, there are few robust results and established findings to guide decisions about the commissioning or the management of services.[37] Palliative care is a complex 'intervention'; it depends on the organization of care, the primary/secondary care interface and the interactions with community care. In addition, the outcomes of care that palliative care aims to achieve are complex, and based mainly on improving the quality of life of both patients and their families and carers. Quality of life is a concept which is hard to measure, particularly in palliative care where patients are often too ill to complete questionnaires or be interviewed, and longitudinal follow-up is difficult.

It is only by using systematic reviews that all the available evidence can be summarized without bias. They fulfil an important role at both extremes of the research process: as definitive summaries and as stimuli for new or further work. The reviews carried out so far point to a dearth of robust research in palliative care, most likely due to the relative infancy of the speciality and the patient population. To continue improving care, research is needed on more patients, across settings, and using similar outcomes to assess effectiveness. Carrying out multicentre studies should be the way forward for research in palliative care.

References

1 Teagarden, J.R. (1989) Meta-analysis: whither narrative review? *Pharmacotherapy*, 9: 274–84.
2 Gotzche, P.C. (1987) Reference bias in reports of drug trials. *British Medical Journal*, 295: 654–6.

3 Mulrow, C.D. (1987) The medical review article: state of the science. *Annals of Internal Medicine*, 166: 485–8.

4 Cooper, H.M. and Rosenthal, R. (1980) Statistical versus traditional procedures for summarising research findings. *Psychological Bulletin*, 87: 442–9.

5 Chalmers, T.C., Prank, C.S. and Reitman, D. (1990) Minimising the three stages of publication bias. *Journal of the American Medical Association*, 263: 139–295.

6 Librach, S.L. and Rapson, L.M. (1988) The use of transcutaneous electrical nerve stimulation (TENS) for the relief of pain in palliative care. *Palliative Medicine*, 2: 15–20.

7 Reeve, J., Menon, C. and Corabian, P. (1995) *Transcutaneous Electrical Nerve Stimulation (TENS): A Technology Assessment*. Ottawa: Canadian Coordinating Office for Health Technology Assessment.

8 Beattie, G., Leonard, R. and Smyth, J. (1989) Bowel obstruction in ovarian carcinoma: a retrospective study and review of the literature. *Palliative Medicine*, 3: 275–80.

9 Farais-Eisner, R., Young, K. and Berek, J. (1994) Bowel obstruction in ovarian cancer. *Seminar of Surgical Oncology*, 10: 268–75.

10 Oxman, A.D. and Ouyatt, G.M. (1993) The science of reviewing research. *Annals of the New York Academy of Science*, 703: 125–31.

11 NHS Centre for Reviews and Dissemination (1996) *Undertaking Systematic Reviews of Research on Effectiveness: CRD Guidelines for Those Carrying Out or Commissioning Reviews*, Report 4. York: NHS Centre for Reviews and Dissemination, University of York.

12 Chalmers, I. and Altman, D.G. (1995) *Systematic Reviews*. London: BMJ Publishing.

13 Chalmers, I. (1993) The Cochrane collaboration: preparing, maintaining and disseminating systematic reviews of the effects of health care. *Annals of the New York Academy of Science*, 703: 156–63.

14 NHS Centre for Reviews and Dissemination (1996) Op. cit.

15 Chalmers, I. and Altman, D.G. (1995) Op. cit.

16 Chalmers, I. (1993) Op. cit.

17 Viola, R., Wells, G. and Peterson, J. (1997) The effects of fluid status and fluid therapy on the dying: a systematic review. *Journal of Palliative Care*, 13: 41–52.

18 Cancer Guidance Subgroup of the Clinical Outcomes Group (1997) *Improving Outcomes in Colorectal Cancer – The Manual*. Leeds: NHS Executive.

19 Cancer Guidance Subgroup of the Clinical Outcomes Group (1997) *Improving Outcomes in Colorectal Cancer – The Research Evidence*. Leeds: NHS Executive.

20 Cancer Guidance Subgroup of the Clinical Outcomes Group (1998) *Improving Outcomes in Lung Cancer: The Manual*. Leeds: NHS Executive.

21 Cancer Guidance Subgroup of the Clinical Outcomes Group (1998) *Improving Outcomes in Lung Cancer: The Research Evidence*. Leeds: NHS Executive.

22 Audit Commission (1993) *What Seems To Be the Matter?* London: HMSO.

23 NHS Centre for Reviews and Dissemination (1996) Op. cit.

24 Chalmers, I. (1993) Op. cit.

25 Dickersin, K., Scherer, R. and Lefebvre, J.C. (1994) Identifying relevant studies for systematic reviews. *British Medical Journal*, 309: 1286–91.

26 Greenhalgh, T. (1997) Searching the literature, in *How to Read a Paper*. London: BMJ Publishing.
27 NHS Centre for Reviews and Dissemination (1996) Op. cit.
28 Rinck, C.G., Geertrudis, A.M., Kleijnen, J. *et al.* (1997) Methodologic issues in effectiveness research on palliative cancer care: a systematic review. *Journal of Clinical Oncology*, 15: 1697–707.
29 www.bmj.com
30 www.oup.co.uk/pubmed/
31 www.cochrane.co.uk
32 NHS Centre for Reviews and Dissemination (1996) Op. cit.
33 Moher, D., Jadad, A.R., Nichol, G. *et al.* (1995) Assessing the quality of randomised controlled trials: an annotated bibliography of scales and checklists. *Controlled Clinical Trials*, 16: 62–73.
34 Schulz, K.F., Chalmers, I., Hayes, R.I. and Altman, D. (1995) Empirical evidence of bias: dimensions of methodological quality associated with estimates of treatment effects in controlled trials. *Journal of the American Medical Association*, 273: 408–12.
35 Oxman, A. (ed.) (1995) Preparing and maintaining systematic reviews, in *Cochrane Collaboration Handbook, Section VI*. Oxford: Cochrane Collaboration.
36 Wiffen, P. (1998) Evidence-based care at the end of life. *Palliative Medicine*, 12: 1–3.
37 Bosanquet, N., Killbery, E., Salisbury, C. *et al.* (1997) *Appropriate and Cost Effective Models of Service Delivery in Palliative Care*. London: Department of Primary Health Care and General Practice, Imperial School of Medicine at St Mary's.

Acknowledgement

Hearn, J., Feuer, D., Higginson, I.J. and Sheldon, T. (1999) Systematic reviews. *Palliative Medicine*, 13: 75–80.

Survey research in palliative care using bereaved relatives*

JULIA M. ADDINGTON-HALL
AND MARK McCARTHY

Introduction

It is increasingly recognized within the NHS that it is important to know what the consumers of services – patients themselves – think about the services provided. In palliative care, particular emphasis is put on the importance of seeing patients and their families as partners in the care process who, wherever possible, should be enabled to make choices about the care they receive. It is, therefore, especially appropriate that the views of patients and their families should be sought when collecting information on the quality or appropriateness of palliative care.

Whose views to collect: those of the patients or families?

Asking patients for their views of the services they receive in the last days and weeks of life is not without difficulties. It can be intrusive to ask patients in their last weeks of life to complete a questionnaire or to be interviewed. Many are too ill to participate by the time they are receiving palliative care services. For instance, 35 per cent of a group of cancer patients with a life expectancy of less than a year died before they could be interviewed.[1] This means that any survey of patients is likely to be unrepresentative – it will include only those patients well enough to take part. It can be difficult to

---

* This is a slightly edited version of the original paper.

ask patients who do not know or acknowledge their diagnosis or prognosis about their experience of palliative care without raising concerns that this will inappropriately alert them to the nature of their illness. Again, this means that patients included in a survey of palliative care are likely to be unrepresentative of all patients receiving these services. Patients may be reluctant to criticize their care, despite reassurances of confidentiality. They may be concerned that their care may be adversely affected if staff get to hear of their criticisms, or may feel that any complaints are a sign of ingratitude. Many patients, particularly those dying of causes other than cancer, die without having been recognized as dying or receiving palliative care. Patient surveys on palliative care exclude these patients and therefore give an incomplete picture of dying.

Although there are several examples of studies which have successfully sought the views of dying people[2-5] it is often more feasible to collect information from relatives about the quality of care provided in a district or by a palliative care service. Interviewing relatives before the patient's death can, however, present some of the same problems as those found when interviewing the patients themselves – it can be difficult to get a representative sample, it may seem intrusive, and relatives may be reluctant to criticize doctors and nurses on whom the patient's comfort depends. An alternative approach which overcomes many of these problems is to talk to relatives after the death of the patient. This has the advantage that a representative sample of deaths in a particular palliative care unit or health district can be included and information can be collected on the whole period leading up to the death. This approach is not without its drawbacks. There are dangers in treating relatives' views as if they accurately represent those of the patients themselves. Even before bereavement, relatives' views of symptom control and service satisfaction are likely to differ from patients' views. For instance, patients have been found to give pain significantly lower ratings than their relatives.[6] Bereaved relatives' views of care will be influenced by bereavement and may differ from their own views before the patient's death. Negative memories come to mind more readily at times of sadness and this may lead to relatives putting more weight on times when things went wrong than on times when care was good. Little is known about the effects of bereavement on how care before the patient's death is remembered and judged. Equally, little is known about how this is influenced by time from death, although the number and extent of differences have been shown to be small in responses to questions on symptoms, need for help and care received, between interviews conducted three and nine months after the death.[7] Some people feel that bereaved people will be distressed by being reminded of the death, and that consequently it is not ethical to ask their views of patient care. However, experience from several large studies which have interviewed bereaved people suggests that the vast majority appreciate the opportunity to talk about the deceased.[8]

Examples of successful surveys of bereaved relatives

There are several examples of interview surveys of bereaved relatives which have shed light on local service provision. For example, 80 bereaved relatives of cancer patients were interviewed in a study carried out in one large district general hospital and results showed that symptom control was a major problem, that the existing community services were inadequate to enable all patients to be at home when desired, and that improvements were needed in the care of dying patients on acute wards.[9] In another study, 37 lay carers of patients in a hospice were interviewed after bereavement.[10] Although most lay carers were satisfied, they were less satisfied with care from community nurses and GPs than from hospice staff, and a minority had had little contact with hospice staff and were dissatisfied with information they had received. Criticisms about communication with professionals were also reported in an interview survey of 106 bereaved relatives of people dying in one health district, as were inadequate symptom control and a lack of bereavement support.[11] Each of these surveys has played an important role in auditing local services by identifying areas where services were failing to meet the needs of patients and relatives.

Interview surveys versus postal questionnaires

Surveys which collect the views of up to 200 people are within the capability of palliative care services, given sufficient planning and adequate resources. The latter will, however, often be a constraint. Because of the need to employ interviewers and to cover their travelling expenses, which may be considerable for palliative care services with large catchment areas, interview surveys are costly. They also require considerable resources and expertise for data entry and processing, analysis and interpretation. An alternative is to use self-completion questionnaires which can be mailed to bereaved relatives.

These are considerably cheaper than interviews, need fewer trained staff to administer and analyse, and remove any danger of interviewer bias. However, postal questionnaires have a number of disadvantages – there is no opportunity for clarification, any ambiguities in answers, or for exploring the reasons respondents hold the views they do. There is also no guarantee that the questionnaire will be completed by the most appropriate person and no way of checking this. For these reasons it has been claimed that an interview will always be better than a self-completed questionnaire in obtaining sensitive information accurately. However, Fitzpatrick[12] has argued that there is no reason why a carefully developed self-completion questionnaire should be as second best as this suggests. There is little experience so far in using postal questionnaires with bereaved people and it is not clear that they would find completing a questionnaire acceptable – they may prefer a face-to-face interview in which they have the opportunity to discuss their concerns and to talk about the deceased.[13] Questionnaires which are seen as invasive or insensitive are unlikely to be returned. It is more difficult to follow up non-responders in a postal survey – interviewers may be able to track down someone if, as is common after bereavement, they have moved but there is no way of doing this with a postal survey. Response rates may therefore be lower than in an interview survey. The question of whether to conduct a postal or interview survey has no straightforward answer and will depend largely upon the resources available.

Questions to consider before starting a survey of bereaved relatives

Regardless of which approach is taken a number of questions need to be considered before beginning such a study.

1 How can relatives be selected so that they are representative of relatives of patients using the service?
2 What are the aims of the exercise? What aspects of the service is it concerned with? Which of these are essential to cover and which could be left out if the questionnaire or interview schedule becomes too long?
3 Is it possible to use existing questionnaires such as that used in the Regional Study of Care for the Dying (RSCD), or questions from them? If new questions are needed, have books on questionnaire design been consulted and/or expert advice sought? Have the questions been piloted to ensure they are acceptable, mean what the investigator thinks, and cover issues the respondents think are important? Have the reliability and validity of the questions been considered?
4 Do additional items of information such as the relationship of the deceased to the relative need to be collected to help in the interpretation of the results?
5 How is the information going to be handled once it is collected? Will it be coded and entered on a computer? If so, how and by whom? What computer software will be used?
6 How will the information be analysed? Are statistics going to be used and, if so, which? Is advice on this needed?
7 Has adequate time been allowed? Are there adequate resources, both in terms of money and people?
8 Is ethical committee approval needed? Should local GPs be informed? Does the study need to be registered under the Data Protection Act?
9 How will the results of this survey be fed back to the palliative care services? What is the mechanism for ensuring that action is taken, if necessary?

It is easy to underestimate the time needed to locate and interview people or to send out questionnaires and reminders, the resources needed to analyse the information collected, and the skills needed to interpret the results. Remember that useful information can be obtained from a small exploratory survey, as long as those included are representative of the relatives of patients using the service. Consider also whether a quantitative survey involving numbers and data analysis is really needed – could the service's requirements be met by a descriptive study in which the views of relatives are collated and described but not coded for statistical analysis? It is important not to undertake a survey of relatives without considering carefully the aims of the survey, the resources available and what advice is needed and from whom it can be gained. There are a number of good references on survey design and questionnaire development[14–16] and it is recommended that some of these are consulted at the planning stage of the study in order to help prevent the investigator from drowning under an over-ambitious project or designing one which produces misleading results.

What action will result from the survey?

One of the risks of asking relatives for their views of palliative care services is that they will not always give the answers the staff expected or ones which the staff find easy to accept. At times, this may lead to a temptation to ignore the results or to find reasons why the answers are biased or misleading. Again, this makes it important for the study to be designed and executed in a way that minimizes bias and maximizes the amount of confidence that can be placed in its findings. Another common temptation is to argue that the problems have been dealt with in the time that has elapsed between the relatives being consulted and the results becoming available and that consequently the results are now irrelevant. Surveys do indeed get out of date and it is important to feed results back as quickly as possible, both to avoid them becoming outdated and to avoid others using this as an argument for ignoring results they do not like. There is no point in asking relatives for their views of services unless these will be listened to, and this means that the ways in which their views will be fed back to the service providers and the mechanisms for acting upon the results should be considered before beginning a survey.

The Regional Study of Care for the Dying

Aims

The Regional Study of Care for the Dying (RSCD), the largest interview survey of bereaved relatives to date in the United Kingdom, was set up at

University College London in 1990 primarily to provide health districts with information to enable them to compare their provision for the dying with that provided by other districts. Other aims included the development of outcome measures for death and bereavement which could be used routinely by district and service providers for quality assurance; the description of the needs of people dying from conditions other than cancer; and the evaluation of the effectiveness of specialist palliative care services. District health authorities (DHAs) in England were invited to take part in the study on the basis that in return for a participation fee the services they provided for the dying would be audited. Twenty districts chose to join the study.

Methods

The methods used in the study built upon those used in two studies by Ann Cartwright who interviewed surviving relatives of a nationally representative sample of deaths in 1969 to describe the last year of life and the adequacy of service provision,[17] and repeated the study in 1987 to see what changes had happened in the intervening years.[18] It was decided to use the same methods and essentially the same interview schedule in the RSCD because these had been shown to be effective, to be capable of detecting change over time and therefore likely to be able to detect differences between districts, and to provide a wealth of valuable information. It would also be possible to compare district results with those of the nationally representative 1987 data. This schedule has also been used as the basis for smaller scale studies.[19,20,21] It has now been simplified and revised for use either in interviews or as a self-completed questionnaire.[22]

Ethical committees

Both the RSCD and the 1987 survey started rather later than anticipated because of delays in obtaining ethical committee approval in participating districts. While some committees were satisfied that the studies presented no major ethical problems and that the proposed study design took adequate account of both the need to be sensitive to bereaved relatives and the need to ensure informed consent was obtained, others expressed considerable alarm at the idea of intruding on the grief of bereaved people. Although permission was finally obtained in all the RSCD districts, two ethical committees approached in the 1987 survey refused permission for the study to go ahead in their areas.[23] Although it is understandable and indeed appropriate that concerns should be expressed about intruding on people's grief, the experience of both studies is that the vast majority of respondents found the opportunity to talk to a sympathetic interviewer about the deceased useful.

Clearly, in such a sensitive area careful consideration needs to be given to ethical considerations. This will include the issue of how best to approach people – in the RSCD a letter was sent to the deceased's address before the interviewer called; while in the 1987 survey the interviewer called without prior warning. The letter enabled people who did not want to take part to telephone the research team immediately, but it also left some relatives concerned about the study or upset by being reminded of their loss without any immediate opportunity to discuss their anxieties with an interviewer. In addition, the letter undoubtedly contributed to the fall in response rate from 80 per cent in 1987 to 69 per cent. Although the reduced response rate may be seen as appropriate – relatives may have felt less able to refuse when approached by an interviewer and therefore were in more danger of feeling coerced to take part – a fall in response rate also has ethical implications; the scientific validity of the study is reduced as the response rate falls and it is unethical to ask people to take part in a study which is of limited validity because of its response rate. Surveys of bereaved relatives do raise difficult ethical issues but, in contrast to the opinion expressed by some ethical committees, the vast majority of respondents seem to find the interview a positive rather than an entirely negative experience.

The sample

Within each district, 270 deaths were sampled randomly from the death certificates of residents aged 16 or over who died in the last quarter of 1990, giving a total sample size of 5378. As cancer patients are the focus of most palliative care services more cancer deaths than non-cancer deaths were sampled. Between seven and 13 months after the deaths, the DHA sent a letter to the address of the deceased to introduce the study and trained interviewers then contacted the address to find the person who knew most about the deceased's last 12 months of life and, if they were willing, to interview them. They succeeded in obtaining interviews for 69 per cent of the sample, and they reported that for 89 per cent of these the person they interviewed had been the most appropriate person to tell them about the last year of life. Wives or husbands were interviewed about 36 per cent of the deceased, children about 30 per cent, other relatives about 16 per cent, friends or neighbours about 9 per cent, and officials about the remaining 10 per cent.

The interview schedule

As deaths were sampled randomly from death certificates, they included the full range of adult deaths from the sudden death of a young person in a motorbike accident to the expected death of an elderly person who had lived in a nursing home for years, had complex medical problems and

---

Box 2.1   The RSCD interview schedule

A   *Contents of the interview schedule*

- Sources of formal and informal care, and respondents' experience of caring for the person who died.
- Symptoms and symptom control.
- Restrictions experienced by the person who died, and the help they received with these.
- Experience of, and satisfaction with, community nursing services, in-patient hospital and hospice care, day centre and GP care.
- Information from, and communication with, health professionals.
- Relatives' experience of bereavement and bereavement care.

B   *Example of question included in interview schedule*

'Altogether, and taking all things into consideration, would you say the care Mrs Jones received, in the year before she died, from the health and social and services was':

excellent	1
good	2
fair	3
poor	4
(other	5)

---

repeated hospital admissions. Consequently the interview schedule, adapted for use from that used by Cartwright and Seale[24] needed to include a wide selection of questions, most of which were relevant only to a sub-section of the sample. The complexity of the schedule, together with the need to be sensitive to the concerns of the bereaved relatives, meant that the survey needed particularly skilful interviews.

Most of the interview schedule was structured and in order to minimize bias arising from the way questions were asked, interviewers were instructed to ask questions exactly as written and in the order they were written. The respondent was asked to choose the most appropriate answer from a number of options given and the interviewer then circled the corresponding number on the schedule, thus reducing the coding needed before responses could be entered on a computer for analysis. A number of open questions were included to help ensure that the respondent had the opportunity to mention issues not otherwise covered, and interviewers were encouraged to record responses to these questions verbatim. Such questions take time and resources to code but can give reports arising from the survey a more 'human' feel, as well as highlighting issues omitted from the schedule because they were not on the investigators' agenda.

Once the schedules were returned to the research team, they were checked for errors and omissions, coded where necessary and entered on a database. These computer files were also carefully checked for errors before data analysis, using the statistical package SPSS-PC. Considerable research, interviewing and computer expertise are required by a study of this size and complexity. However, as already discussed, useful results can also come out of much smaller surveys.

Feedback to districts

The districts who took part in the RSCD did so because they wanted information on how need for, and satisfaction with, their services for the dying compared with that elsewhere. Providing them with feedback was, therefore, one of the main aims of the study. Each district received a comprehensive package of feedback which compared the district's score on each question to that for the study as a whole, for cancer and non-cancer deaths separately. In order to help districts interpret their results the feedback was accompanied by a description of service provision in each district and an explanation of how response bias may have affected the results.

Conclusion

While a large survey will be outside the capabilities of most palliative care services, many will be able to undertake small interview or postal surveys of bereaved relatives of patients who have received their services, given sufficient planning and resources. Relatives can give a valuable perspective on palliative care services and their views can help prevent professionals falling into the trap of providing services they think are required, rather than those which actually are. The difficulties of collecting the views of relatives in a systematic way can seem overwhelming, but the benefits of doing so can greatly outweigh the problems en route.

References

1 Addington-Hall, J.M., MacDonald, L.D., Anderson, H.R. *et al.* (1992) Randomised controlled trial of effects of co-ordinating care for terminally ill cancer patients. *British Medical Journal*, 305: 1317–21.
2 Field, D., Douglas, C., Jagger, C. and Dand, P. (1995) Terminal illness: views of patients and their lay carers. *Palliative Medicine*, 9: 45–54.
3 Higginson, I., Wade, A. and McCarthy, M. (1990) Palliative care: views of patients and their families. *British Medical Journal*, 301: 227–80.
4 Hinton, J. (1994) Can home care maintain an acceptable quality of life for patients with terminal cancer and their relatives? *Palliative Medicine*, 8: 183–96.

 5 Townsend, J., Frank, O.O., Fermont, D. *et al.* (1990) Terminal cancer care and patients' preference for place of death: a prospective study. *British Medical Journal*, 301: 415–17.
 6 Curtis, A.E. and Fernester, J. (1989) Quality of life of oncology hospice patients: a comparison of patients and primary caregivers' reports. *Oncology Nursing Forum*, 16: 49–53.
 7 Cartwright, A., Hockey, L. and Anderson, J.L. (1973) *Life Before Death*. London: Routledge and Kegan Paul.
 8 Cartwright, A. and Seale, C. (1990) *The Natural History of a Survey*. London: King's Fund Centre.
 9 Addington-Hall, J.M., MacDonald, L.D., Anderson, H.R. and Freeling, P. (1991) Dying from cancer: the views of bereaved family and friends about the experience of terminally ill patients. *Palliative Medicine*, 5: 207–14.
10 Field, D., Dand, P., Ahmedzai, S. and Biswas, B. (1992) Care and information received by lay carers of terminally ill patients at the Leicestershire hospice. *Palliative Medicine*, 6: 237–45.
11 Sykes, N.P., Pearson, S.E. and Chell, S. (1992) Quality of care of the terminally ill: the carer's perspective. *Palliative Medicine*, 6: 227–36.
12 Fitzpatrick, R. (1991) Surveys of patient satisfaction: I – Important general considerations. *British Medical Journal*, 302: 887–9.
13 Curtis, A.E. and Fernester, J. (1989) Op. cit.
14 Abramson, J.H. (1990) *Survey Methods in Community Medicine*, 4th edition. London: Churchill Livingstone.
15 Bowling, A. (1998) *Research Methods in Health: Investigating Health and Health Services*. Buckingham: Open University Press.
16 Moser, C. and Kalton, G. (1971) *Survey Methods in Social Investigation*. Aldershot: Gower Publishing Group.
17 Cartwright, A., Hockey, L. and Anderson, J.L. (1973) Op. cit.
18 Cartwright, A. and Seale, C. (1990) Op. cit.
19 Field, D. *et al.* (1992) Op. cit.
20 St Leger, A.S., Schnieden, H. and Walsworth-Bell, J.P. (1992) *Evaluating Health Services' Effectiveness*. Buckingham: Open University Press.
21 Field, D. and McGaughey, J. (1998) An evaluation of palliative care services for cancer patients in the South Health and Social Services Board of Northern Ireland. *Palliative Medicine*, 12: 83–97.
22 Addington-Hall, J.M., Walker, L., Jones, C., Karlsen, S. and McCarthy, M.A. (1998) Randomised controlled trial of postal versus interviewer administration of a questionnaire measuring satisfaction with and use of services received in the year before death. *Journal of Epidemiology and Community Health*, 52: 802–7.
23 Cartwright, A. and Seale, C. (1990) Op. cit.
24 Ibid.

Acknowledgement

Addington-Hall, J. and McCarthy, M. (1993) Survey research in palliative care: using bereaved relatives, in I.J. Higginson (ed.) *Clinical Audit in Palliative Care*. Oxford: Radcliffe Medical Press.

3 How many subjects are needed in a research sample in palliative care?

SARA FAITHFULL

The number of subjects in a trial designed to determine treatment effectiveness is only one element in determining the statistical power of a study. Statistical power refers to the probability that a test of the null hypothesis (which states that there is no difference between the treatments under consideration) will give statistical significance when in fact the null hypothesis is false. Low statistical power can result in an intervention that may be beneficial being disregarded as ineffective, and while researchers are aware of the importance of large samples, many studies have insufficient power to detect differences in treatment groups. This is a common problem in palliative care and is indicative of how difficult it is to collect the relatively large numbers of patients required for treatment effectiveness research.

In clinical research, interest often centres on the difference between treatment and control groups. A major obstacle in hospice and palliative care research is that the pool of available subjects is small, and often varies with different disease states, symptoms and stages of illness. Research in these areas involves multiple variables and complex treatment, the effects of which must by necessity be studies in the ward or clinic rather than in the controlled environment of the laboratory.[1]

In the planning of a study, the researcher is obviously concerned that he will be able to detect true differences in his sample population (Figure 3.1). The testing of whether there is a significant treatment effect can be thought of as comparing how large the differences are between the control and experimental groups.[2] If there is a large variation between the individuals in the different groups the power of the study may be reduced. This is usually overcome by increasing the sample size. This is not the only way of improving the statistical power and several other factors need to be decided before it is possible to determine the sample size.

Figure 3.1 Testing the effectiveness of an intervention. The extent of the difference between the two arms of a study is reflected in how the effect is measured as well as the techniques for analysing that effect

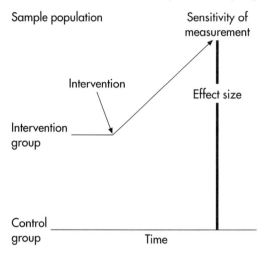

Different errors may occur in a research study. In Type I errors, the researcher concludes that there is a significant difference between samples when in fact there is no such difference. Type II errors occur when the researcher fails to gain statistical significance and concludes that there is no difference when in fact a difference does exist.[3]

The probability of a Type I error occurring is referred to as the α level, and is conventionally set at 1 in 20 (0.05, or 5 per cent). Type II errors have been relatively neglected in treatment effectiveness research but are linked very closely to the sample size. The risk of allowing a truly effective intervention to go undiscovered is therefore increased in small sample studies.[4] The probability of a Type II error occurring is expressed as the β level: if this is set at 0.2 (or 20 per cent) the study will have a power of 0.8 (or 80 per cent).

While sample size is important, it is only one of four factors that increase the statistical power of the study:

- statistical tests – the test itself is one of the factors determining statistical power. Different tests do not necessarily have the same statistical power when they are applied to the same data;
- α level – the level set for α influences the likelihood of statistical significance;
- effect size – the size of the proposed treatment response in the intervention group will have an important influence on the likelihood of attaining statistical significance. The larger the effect, the more probable it is that positive results will be detectable;

- sample size – statistical significance testing is concerned with sampling error, which refers to the expected discrepancies that can be found in a study. The sampling error is greater for smaller studies and almost negligible for very large samples.

The link between statistical power and sample size is so close that many researchers discuss power only as a form of determining the size of the sample required. This emphasis is misplaced as it leaves the impression that it is only a matter of the researcher making the study large enough to be able to test treatment effectiveness,[5] but sample size remains only one of four factors. The challenge in palliative care is keeping adequate power with modest sample sizes.

To decide the numerical values required in a study it is possible to look up the statistical power in tables.[6] The way in which the other three factors influence the sample size is more easily seen by the use of a chart rather than a table. Figure 3.2 gives an indication of how the effect size influences sample size. At any given sample size below 200, statistical power increases dramatically with increases in effect size. An important aspect of planning any study is thus to explore how effective the proposed intervention is and how sensitive the design of the study is in picking up this effect.

In studies of treatment effectiveness there has been a long history of large studies, for example multicentre clinical trials. This discourages researchers

Figure 3.2 The relationship between sample size and effect size (ES: effect size)

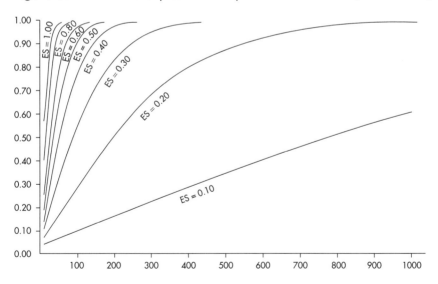

Source: Lipsey, M.W. (1990) *Design Sensitivity.* Thousand Oaks, CA: Sage. Reprinted by permission of Sage Publications.

from testing treatment interventions in small sample groups. To illustrate how sample size and treatment effectiveness are interlinked it is helpful to use an example. Thus, a meta-analysis of published clinical research found that researchers reporting a treatment's effectiveness often used small sample sizes.[7] The mean sample size for each arm of a study was 40, making an average sample of 80 in total. A recent analysis of nursing studies found that only 15 per cent of studies had sufficient power for their data analysis.[8]

The majority of health studies were therefore underpowered. If it is assumed that the researcher requires a power of 0.95 ($\beta = 0.05$, $\alpha = 0.05$) and proposes a treatment effect of 18 per cent improvement, the sample size would need to be a minimum of 700 subjects in each group (total 1400). A more modest power of 0.80 ($\beta = 0.20$) would still require a sample of about 400 subjects per group and 800 subjects in total. This highlights the difficulty that researchers can have if the focus is on sample size alone. As can be seen in this example, the effect size has great implications for researchers.

It is possible to increase design sensitivity and hence the statistical power without resorting to large sample studies.[9] The factors that can enhance design sensitivity are illustrated in Table 3.1.

While increasing the sample size is a practical method for increasing statistical power and should be used wherever feasible, it is not always possible for the researcher in palliative care to use this approach. Awareness of alternative strategies can be useful. Issues of design sensitivity are often widely neglected in planning research, but treatment effectiveness research is often designed at such a low level of sensitivity that many studies have

Table 3.1   Factors that work to increase design sensitivity

Treatment	1	A strong treatment effect
	2	Uniform application of treatment
Sample	1	A population that is similar in characteristics
Measurement	1	Tools sensitive to the changes expected
	2	Fine measurements rather than global scores
	3	The ability to explore both mild and severe sensations
	4	Measurement that is unresponsive to irrelevant changes
	5	Consistency in measurement procedures
	6	Timing of measurement to coincide with the peak response
	7	Measurement of effects closer to the intervention rather than longer term effects
Analysis	1	Use of a larger α for significance testing
	2	One directional hypothesis test
	3	Significance tests for graduated scores

little chance of detecting the effects they plan to investigate.[10] It does not make sense to design a study that will fail to gain statistical results. If large samples are not possible then exploration of how to increase effect size, α level and statistical tests are well worth exploring.[11]

References

1 Lipsey, M.W. (1990) *Design Sensitivity: Statistical Power for Experimental Research.* London: Sage.
2 Beck, C.T. (1994) Achieving statistical power through research design sensitivity. *Journal of Advanced Nursing*, 20: 912–16.
3 Burns, N. and Groves, S.K. (1987) *The Practice of Nursing Research: Conduct Critique and Utilization.* Philadelphia, PA: WB Saunders.
4 Beck, C.T. (1994) Op. cit.
5 Kraemer, H.C. and Thiemann, S. (1987) *How Many Subjects? Statistical Power Analysis in Research.* London: Sage.
6 Cohen, J. (1988) *Statistical Power Analysis for the Behavioral Sciences.* Hillsdale, NJ: Lawrence Erlbaum Associates.
7 Lipsey, M.W. (1990) Op. cit.
8 Polit, D. and Sherman, R. (1990) Statistical power in nursing research. *Nursing Research*, 39: 365–9.
9 Beck, C.T. (1994) Op. cit.
10 Lipsey, M.W. (1990) Op. cit.
11 Beck, C.T. (1994) Op. cit.

Acknowledgement

Faithfull, S. (1996) How many subjects are needed in a research sample in palliative care? *Palliative Medicine*, 10: 259–61.

Placebo-controlled trials in palliative care: the argument for

JANET R. HARDY

> A placebo is an intervention designed to simulate medical therapy, but not believed (by the investigator or clinician) to be a specific therapy for the target condition.[1]
>
> A placebo effect is a change in a patient's illness attributable to the symbolic import of a treatment rather than a specific pharmacological or physiological property or, non-specific effects.[2]

Effective treatment

One of the strongest arguments for the use of placebo-controlled trials in palliative care is to counter what is seen as one of the strongest arguments against, i.e. that 'a placebo control in a clinical trial is unethical if a proven therapy already exists'.[3] This argument is theoretically strengthened by the *Declaration of Helsinki* which states that 'every patient – including those of a control group, if any – should be assured of the best proven diagnostic and therapeutic method'.[4]

The problem is that many, if not most of the 'standard' treatments in palliative care have never been proven to be effective and their use is based on anecdote and physician preference. There are many examples of this, including anticonvulsants and/or anti-arrhythmics in cancer-related neuropathic pain, antiemetics in opioid-induced nausea, corticosteroids in intestinal obstruction, non-steroidal anti-inflammatory drugs (NSAIDs) in chronic cancer-related bone pain, and thioridazine for night sweats.

This situation applies not only to palliative care. The presumption that if a treatment is widely used it must have some benefit has been shaken not only by reports that many common treatments have no supporting evidence of effectiveness, but also by trials that have overturned some common beliefs,[5] for example flecainide after myocardial infarction, corticosteroids for optic neuritis, blood letting, gastric freezing for ulcers, radical mastectomy and routine tonsillectomy. It is no longer acceptable to use a particular treatment because an individual physician believes that it is in the patient's best interest. As stated by Eddy,[6] 'the credibility of clinical judgment has been severely challenged by observations of wide variations in clinical practice, inappropriate care, and practitioner uncertainty'. The classic palliative care example of this is in the management of neuropathic pain; physicians cannot even agree on whether or not this is opioid sensitive, let alone on the role of anticonvulsants/antidepressants and other drugs.

The comment is often made that 'I don't need a trial to prove that our drugs work'; 'I know they work from everyday experience.' One would query, however, whether most practitioners in the field know how powerful the placebo effect or non-specific effects of their drugs are likely to be.

The placebo effect

'Symptoms, illness and their changes over time reflect complex interactions between anatomical and neurophysical processes on the one hand and cognitive-behavioral and environmental factors on the other.'[7] There is thus a large subjective component inherent in many of the symptoms and illnesses we treat.

There is also an important time factor. This is known as 'natural history and regression to the mean'.[8] Most acute and some chronic pain problems resolve on their own, irrespective of treatment. Patients with chronic conditions typically have fluctuating symptoms and seek medical care when symptoms are at their worst. Thus the next change is likely to be an improvement (a regression to the mean). An example of this is opioid-induced nausea and vomiting. This is often a transient phenomenon that subsides after a few days.[9] Patients are likely to ask for antiemetics when their discomfort is at its worst. It is thus difficult to say whether any subsequent improvement is related to the anti-emetic or whether it reflects the natural course of the condition which was likely to have improved anyway.

There are placebo effects involved whenever the patient and clinician perceive a treatment as being effective. These effects are potent, and can lead to erroneous claims of efficacy.[10] Those of us who believed strongly in the beneficial effects of nebulized morphine for the palliation of breathlessness tended to get good results when offering this 'treatment' to patients. Those of us who were more sceptical about its benefits tended to have less impressive results. Now that several trials have shown nebulized morphine to be no more effective than placebo, one must wonder how much our initial enthusiasm swayed our earlier experience.

It is essential for all involved in the giving of palliative care to understand the extent to which placebo effects can account for improvements observed in clinical practice. Probably the most striking example of this is in the underestimation of the non-specific or placebo effects in many pain treatment and research situations. The placebo response to pain is often much greater than the widely accepted figure of 30 per cent. A review of placebo effects in studies of medical and surgical treatments for painful conditions subsequently shown to be totally ineffective or 'sham treatment' gave an average response of 70 per cent with a 100 per cent response rate in some cases.[11] Examples include 100 per cent improvements in angina pectoris following both internal mammary artery ligation and skin excision only and an 83 per cent excellent or good improvement in the pain associated with herpes simplex infections treated by photodynamic inactivation treatment (treatments subsequently found to be no better than placebo in controlled trials).[12]

Efforts to identify personality and other characteristics that predict for placebo response have had little success,[13] but patient expectations of treatment effects clearly influence their responses.[14] Asthmatic patients given isotonic saline had increases or decreases in airways resistance according to what they were told to expect.[15] When we discuss treatment plans with patients we are much more likely to say 'This will help your pain' rather than 'This has never been proven to be of any benefit but let's try it anyway!'

There is some evidence that placebo response is strongest in patients who are anxious, dependent and noncritical.[16,17] Palliative care patients who have 'lost their fight against cancer' have every reason to be anxious, frightened and dependent, often having lost control of their lives and treatment, and therefore may well be those who one would expect to respond to placebo. Similarly one might hope that palliative care practitioners are likely to be caring, considerate and prepared to devote time! The providers of warmth, friendliness, interest, sympathy, empathy, prestige and a positive attitude toward the patient and their treatment are associated with positive effects of placebos as well as active treatments.[18] Physician attention, interest and concern in a healing setting all contribute to the non-specific benefits of healing.[19]

There is also a factor known as 'obsequious bias'. When a patient appreciates the efforts of a clinician, a willingness to please (or at least not disappoint) the clinician may cause the patient to minimize symptoms or overestimate recovery.[20]

In summary, as stated by Turner et al.,[21] 'The extent to which patient outcomes after a medical or surgical treatment reflect non-specific treatment effects is unclear in the absence of randomised controlled trials with outcomes assessed by persons blind to the patient's treatment.' The double-blind randomized placebo-controlled trial avoids or accommodates all the pitfalls as described above. I would agree with McQuay and Moore[22] that 'the time has come to put an end to the casual use of "effectiveness" as an easy way out – you say that it's effective, then prove it!'

Justifications

Equipoise

The classic equipoise requirement for ethical randomization is in the comparison of two treatments, neither of which is known to be superior.[23] When there is no evidence that drug x is better than placebo, and we *do* know that the placebo effect is so powerful, there can be no argument against the use of a placebo-controlled trial. It could be said that palliative care has 'shot itself in the foot'. No one is postulating a placebo-controlled trial of a new analgesic alone in morphine-sensitive pain, but because so many of the 'treatments' in palliative care have never been subject to study, there is no proof of their effectiveness and therefore no argument against a placebo-controlled trial when evaluating them. Once again, this applies not only to palliative care, but to many specialities; it is estimated that 80–90 per cent of all treatments in common usage have not been adequately evaluated in controlled studies.[24]

The statement was recently made in an argument against placebo that 'when an effective treatment exists and then a new one comes along, it is only common sense to ask whether the new treatment beats the old – who cares whether the new treatment is more or less effective than nothing?'[25] I care, if the old treatment has never been proven to be any better than placebo. One is then in danger of deceiving the patient and subjecting them to the possibility of unwarranted toxicity, let alone the health service to unjustified expense.

Gold standard

The gold standard in clinical research is the randomized placebo-controlled double-blind clinical trial.[26] Placebo-controlled trials offer the greatest scientific rigour for assessing the efficacy of a drug.[27] They have become the standard scientific strategy for determining the efficacy of therapy because they allow for all the problems as described above. Many old treatments have been ushered in during periods when the threshold for sufficient evidence was much lower.[28] Different burdens of proof have evolved for new versus old treatments and the controlled clinical trial is now an essential component for assessing interventions.[29,30] In these times of resource rationalization it has been asked if medical decisions not supported by randomized controlled trials will still be supported.[31]

Proof is scientifically strongest if data comes from trials that compare new drugs with placebo, with interventions given in a double-blind fashion and in random order. 'Medicine the science is gradually replacing medicine the art.'[32]

'Too hard? – too bad'

It is generally acknowledged that it is very difficult to accrue the numbers of patients necessary to do a randomized trial in palliative care.[33,34] We have abandoned three such trials because of poor patient accrual.[35] The patients under study are often very ill and many have 'trial fatigue'. Their carers may be unwilling to expose them to what might be seen as further experimentation.[36] But is this a reason to excuse palliative care from the rigours of proper research?[37] What is the excuse for not doing large multicentre studies in palliative care? Pharmaceutical companies have shown that this is 'doable' in studies of new analgesics.[38] Studies in palliative care may be more difficult than standard placebo-controlled studies of new anti-cancer drugs in established research centres, but not impossible and there is at least one advantage. In studies which have time to an event as the primary endpoint (for example, time to correction of hypercalcaemia, time to discharge or death) statistical power depends on the number of events. Such events happen relatively quickly in palliative care and hence studies in palliative care can be of shorter duration. This is very different to a study of adjuvant therapy in breast cancer in which survival over many years is being measured.

Research is not necessarily bad for patients

There are a number of studies that compare outcome of patients treated within clinical trials with that of a similar population of patients not entered into research protocols – most of these studies suggest that patients fare better if treated in the context of a properly conducted trial,[39] presumably because they have closer supervision and more frequent assessments.

If palliative care is to be taken seriously as a medical speciality in its own right it has to be seen to be able to justify what it does and show that it can perform high-quality research. Evidence-based care is becoming more of a necessity than a buzz-word. Surely our main aim must be to do the very best for our patients, and if this means subjecting them to the highest standards of clinical research – so be it!

References

1 Brody, H. (1985) Placebo effect: an examination of Grunbaum's definition, in L. White, B. Tursky and G.E. Schwartz (eds) *Placebo, Theory Research and Mechanisms*. New York, NY: Guilford Press.

2 Ibid.
3 Taubes, G. (1995) Use of placebo controls in clinical trials disputed. *Science*, 267: 25–6.
4 World Medical Association (1989) *Declaration of Helsinki Fernay-Voltaire.* World Medical Association.
5 Eddy, D.M. (1993) Three battles to watch in the 1990s. Clinical decision making. *Journal of the American Medical Association*, 270: 520–6.
6 Ibid.
7 Turner, J.A., Deyo, R.A., Loeser, J.D., Von Korff, M. and Fordyce, W.E. (1994) The importance of placebo effects in pain treatment and research. *Journal of the American Medical Association*, 271: 1609–14.
8 Ernst, E. and Resch, K.L. (1995) Concept of true and perceived placebo effects. *British Medical Journal*, 311: 551–3.
9 Twycross, R. (1994) Oral morphine in *Pain Relief in Advanced Cancer*, Ch. 16. Edinburgh: Churchill Livingstone.
10 Eddy, D.M. (1993) Op. cit.
11 Ibid.
12 Ibid.
13 Shapiro, A.K. and Shapiro, E. (1984) Patient provider relationships and the placebo effect, in J.D. Matarazzo, S.M. Weiss, J.A. Herd, N.E. Miller and S.M. Weiss (eds) *Behavioral Health: A Handbook of Health Enhancement and Disease Prevention*. New York, NY: Wiley–Interscience.
14 Eddy, D.M. (1993) Op. cit.
15 Luparello, T., Leist, N., Lourie, C.H. and Sweet, P. (1970) The interaction of psychologic stimuli and pharmacologic agents on airway reactivity in asthmatic subjects. *Psychosomatic Medicine*, 32: 509–13.
16 Shapiro, A.K. and Shapiro, E. (1984) Op. cit.
17 Chaput de Saintonge, D.M. and Herxheimer, A. (1994) Harnessing placebo effects in health care. *Lancet*, 344: 995–8.
18 Ernst, E. and Resch, K.L. (1995) Op. cit.
19 Chaput de Saintonge, D.M. and Herxheimer, A. (1994) Op. cit.
20 Guyatt, G., Sackett, D., Wayne, T.D. *et al.* (1986) Determining optimal therapy – randomized trials in individual patients. *New England Journal of Medicine*, 314: 889–92.
21 Turner, J.A. *et al.* (1994) Op. cit.
22 McQuay, H. and Moore, A. (1994) Need for rigorous assessment of palliative care. *British Medical Journal*, 309: 1315–16.
23 Freedman, B. (1987) Equipoise and the ethics of clinical research. *New England Journal of Medicine*, 317: 141–5.
24 Eddy, D.M. (1993) Op. cit.
25 Rothman, K.J. (1996) Placebo mania. *British Medical Journal*, 313: 3–4.
26 Jones, B., Jarvis, P., Lewis, J.A. and Ebbutt, A.F. (1996) Trials to assess equivalence: the importance of rigorous methods. *British Medical Journal*, 313: 36–9.
27 Dollery, C.T. (1979) A bleak outlook for placebos (and for science). *European Journal of Clinical Pharmacology*, 15: 219–21.
28 Ibid.
29 Ibid.

30 Rothman, K.J. and Michels, K.B. (1994) Sounding board: the continuing unethical use of placebo controls. *New England Journal of Medicine*, 331: 394–8.
31 McQuay and Moore (1994) Op. cit.
32 Collier, J. (1995) Confusion over use of placebos in clinical trials. *British Medical Journal*, 311: 821–2.
33 McWhinney, I.R.M., Bass, M.J. and Donner, A. (1994) Evaluation of a palliative care service: problems and pitfalls. *British Medical Journal*, 309: 1340–2.
34 Faithfull, S. (1996) How many subjects are needed in a research sample in palliative care? *Palliative Medicine*, 10: 259–61.
35 Ling, J. and Hardy, J. (1996) The failure of placebo controlled trials of bisphosphonates in bone pain [Abstract]. *Palliative Care Research Forum*, Coventry, November.
36 Ling, J. and Penn, K. (1996) Recruitment figures may be low [Abstract]. *Palliative Medicine*, 10: 68–9.
37 Ibid.
38 Ahmedzai, S. and Brooks, D.J. (1996) Transdermal fentanyl versus oral morphine in the treatment of cancer pain [Abstract]. *Palliative Medicine*, 10: 60–1.
39 Slevin, M., Mossman, J., Bowling, A., Leonard, R. and Steward, W. *et al.* (1995) Volunteers or victims: patients' view of randomised cancer clinical trials. *British Journal of Cancer*, 71: 1270–4.

Acknowledgements

I wish to acknowledge the comments of members of the South Thames Palliative Care Research Group which were taken into consideration when preparing this manuscript.

Reprinted from Hardy, J.R. (1997) Placebo-controlled trials in palliative care: the argument for. *Palliative Medicine*, 11: 415–18.

5 Placebo-controlled trials in palliative care: the argument against

STEPHEN R. KIRKHAM AND J. ABEL

Introduction

It has been suggested that the double-blind placebo-controlled randomized clinical trial is the gold standard for the investigation of new treatments.[1] It would neither be appropriate nor even possible to argue that the inclusion of placebo preparations is inappropriate in many of these studies, although it is worth remembering that the randomized placebo-controlled clinical trial is only one way of collecting evidence. Within evidence-based medicine Gray describes five levels of strength of evidence.[2] His list is reproduced in Table 5.1, and it is worth noting that the word 'placebo' does not occur. Placebo controls should therefore not be considered to be a prerequisite for scientific validity, even under the most stringent definitions.

Within the field of cancer treatment, new cytotoxic agents, which are some of the most expensive modern drugs, are evaluated in phase II studies by comparison with historical controls, and in phase III studies by comparison with established treatments.[3] Placebo controls are not considered mandatory.

As palliative care physicians, we need to ask ourselves whether it is anyway appropriate that we limit our prescribing solely to drugs which have been shown to be effective in placebo-controlled trials. While these trials can give good evidence of the pharmacodynamic effect, they are not the only way of assessing how well a drug works.

It is clear that there are historical, practical and ethical difficulties which arise if one stipulates that all treatments which are used in the field of palliative care should be regarded as being of doubtful efficacy, unless they have been subjected to a formal placebo-controlled trial.

Table 5.1   The five strengths of evidence

Type	Strength of evidence
I	Strong evidence from at least one systematic review of multiple well-designed randomized controlled trials
II	Strong evidence from at least one properly designed randomized controlled trial of appropriate size
III	Evidence from well-designed trials without randomization, single group pre-post, cohort, time series or matched case-control studies
IV	Evidence from well-designed non-experimental studies from more than one centre or research group
V	Opinions of respected authorities, based on clinical evidence, descriptive studies or reports of expert committees

Source: Gray, J.A.M. (1997) Evidence-based Healthcare. London: Churchill Livingstone.

Difficulties of placebo-controlled trials

The use of placebo-controlled trials has only grown up in the past 30 years or so.[4] Most of the treatments which were widely accepted before that time have not been subject to such evaluation. Frequently, no one would even suggest that they were, since their efficacy is so obvious. With the possible exception of neuropathic pain, one does not need to conduct a placebo-controlled trial of morphine to discover that it is an effective analgesic, nor of corticosteroids to discover that they provide symptomatic improvement in many patients with cerebral tumour.

Application of strict scientific method in humans is at the very least extremely difficult. We are creatures of chaos, resembling complex weather systems more than complex machines, and altering one variable may well cause unexpected results. Medicine is not like experimental physics: we are unable to isolate a single variable and watch the effect of its changing. We therefore need to use a variety of methods to assess the usefulness of our interventions; it would be unrealistic to suppose that all problems could be solved with one experimental technique.

It is well known that it is difficult to carry out trials in palliative care. There are numerous problems: the patients may be too ill to complete questionnaires; there may be a high attrition rate; and there may not be a sufficient number of patients to achieve a significant result in a drug study in which large numbers of subjects are needed to demonstrate efficacy.[5] Even in the interpretation of such studies it is worth remembering that most trials which reach negative results are never published. If statistical significance is taken at the 0.05 level, 5 per cent of trials will therefore show a false-positive (Type I error) result. Relying solely on published trials before deciding what to prescribe may therefore not be as secure as we might imagine.

It has been accepted in the past[6,7] that the amount of relief obtained from placebo is around one-third of the maximum possible, and that one-third of patients respond to placebo. If this were reliably so, we could isolate the placebo element in drug trials to give a good estimate of efficacy. However, this is not the case, as good studies have shown.[8] There is instead considerable variation in the figure, implying that placebo-controlled trials may not be as reliable as might be expected.

It is part of the whole licensing procedure for new drugs that they should be evaluated fastidiously, both from the point of view of efficacy and toxicity. Much of the demand for such rigour followed the thalidomide disaster, although it has been pointed out that even stringent modern toxological evaluation would probably not have predicted or prevented such a catastrophe being repeated if thalidomide had only just been discovered.[9]

The expense of mounting a placebo-controlled trial (which may be considerable) is taken into account in the pricing structure for a new preparation. Where a drug is already available with an established pricing structure, as often applies in palliative care, the research may simply be impossible to fund.

It is entirely true that many, and indeed most, of the drug treatments used in palliative care have not formally been proven to be effective by randomized trial. Well-known examples where controversy exists include the use of nonsteroidal anti-inflammatory drugs (NSAIDs) for bone pain, which may be effective in about 80 per cent of patients[10] or largely ineffective,[11] depending on one's point of view; and the use of metoclopramide in intestinal obstruction, which has both been promoted as the anti-emetic of choice[12] and said to be contra-indicated.[13]

We suggest that if research were proposed to examine either of these two questions, the question as to how best to carry it out should be approached simultaneously from three different viewpoints. These relate to the need to satisfy in turn the requirements of members of a local research ethics committee who will be giving their permission for the research to take place, editors of specialist journals who might be publishing the results, and clinical staff in palliative care, who will be applying the work to the needs of their patients.

Members of research ethics committees need to know that the research which is proposed will not cause any harm to the patients who will be studied; they must also take into account its impact on society at large, but this is inevitably a secondary consideration. Thus, the ethical imperative of proving whether a treatment is effective from the point of view of society at large does not outweigh the ethical imperative of 'I do my best for my patients', whether that is in a clinical or a research setting. As such, however urgent the need to find an answer to the problem, giving a placebo to a patient who is mortally ill and who is vomiting is unlikely to receive ethical approval.

Editors will look for clarity of thought and design within an ethically accepted framework. A paper which shows that a drug which is licensed for use in the management of pain or of vomiting is more effective than placebo in treating these symptoms merely reports something that is already well established, and is unlikely to be accepted for publication unless it shows something unexpected.

Clinicians want a study which gives a clear result, which will be of everyday use. The notion that a particular treatment is statistically more effective than placebo only goes half way in fulfilling this criterion, since the question has a single tail – does the drug work? We will never prescribe placebo, so ultimately the question which needs to be answered is, what is the best treatment?

Even here we need to bear in mind the question of applicability, and the difference between explanatory and pragmatic studies.[14] In an explanatory study, a group of highly selected and uniform subjects is studied, perhaps with the intention of determining not only whether a treatment is effective, but how it works. This kind of study gives good scientific evidence, but it cannot be assumed that it has general clinical applicability. On the other hand, a pragmatic study recruits a disparate group of subjects, and tries to determine whether the treatment will help the 'average' patient.

An example might be made as follows: in studying the effects of corticosteroids in anorexia, an explanatory study might be conducted on normocalcaemic patients with squamous cell carcinoma of the bronchus and anorexia, who have normal scores on the Hospital Anxiety and Depression (HAD) scale. Patients are prescribed the same or varying doses of corticosteroids, and appetite and various biochemical parameters are closely monitored. Good information may be obtained on the aetiology of anorexia in these patients, but this may not apply in patients with ovarian carcinoma. On the other hand, a pragmatic study might be performed, in which, with a few exclusions, all patients attending a clinic with anorexia in association with a malignancy are entered into a study which follows changes in appetite after prescription of corticosteroids.

It is entirely possible that both of these models would follow the randomized placebo-controlled trial model. But for the clinician, the second will have everyday applicability, while the first will tend to encourage further research. Here, a placebo-controlled (explanatory) trial does not provide the answer.

In the first instance of unresolved controversies given above, relating to the usefulness of NSAIDs in bone pain, placebo-controlled trials are unlikely to be helpful simply because they will not mimic the normal clinical situation. Substantial progress could, however, be made by studying patients presenting with bone pain, perhaps uncontrolled on paracetamol and/or weak opioids. Precise evaluation of the nature of their analgesia after they had been randomized to receive either a strong opioid or an NSAID with appropriate rescue analgesia would provide invaluable information with no need to use placebo. In an ideal world this would be conducted as a double-blind trial, in which the two study drugs were identical in appearance. The chances of this being feasible, however, are vanishingly small; an alternative would be to use a double dummy technique, in which the active form of one drug was given with a placebo of the other, so that neither patient nor clinician was aware of the nature of the treatment. The importance of the placebo here is in blinding all parties to the nature of the treatment, not in providing an inactive treatment. At a practical level however, the pharmaceutical companies may be unwilling, and indeed unable, to provide placebo formulations of very well-accepted preparations, and the study would still be valid if it were conducted in an open randomized fashion. In the second example, within a population of obstructed patients, metoclopramide could be compared with another anti-emetic such as methotrimeprazine to determine their effects and toxicity in a group of obstructed patients.

Inevitably, major problems will arise where there is no accepted treatment for a condition. An example here might be weakness: many reports indicate that this is the commonest symptom which afflicts patients with advanced malignant disease,[15] and indeed it may be inevitable, unless death comes unexpectedly early through some other catastrophe. One might think that, if there is no accepted treatment, a placebo-controlled trial would provide the best solution, but difficulties may still arise.

Suppose that it is suggested that such weakness is aggravated by vitamin deficiency, which itself has been aggravated by poor nutritional intake. In a placebo-controlled trial, it would be necessary to seek informed consent from potential subjects, during which process they would be told that they would be given either vitamins or placebo. Realistically, how many patients would be recruited? Of those entering the study, how many would surreptitiously take one form of vitamin or another? Even here, where there is no accepted treatment, it is likely to be more practicable to compare one vitamin preparation with another, preferably with no overlap between the two in terms of constituents. Thus, one might compare a compound vitamin B preparation with another containing vitamins A, C and E.

Placebo effects in a broader context

Our role as clinicians is not limited to the prescription of drugs. We need good diagnostic, therapeutic and communication skills; all of these will influence the results of our interventions. A knowledge of a drug's proven pharmacodynamic properties is only one reason why we choose to prescribe it. We should also be experts in maximizing the placebo effect.[16] This is not merely telling a patient that a drug works; it has been shown that a drug is more effective if the physician believes it works.[17,18] Thus prescribing a particular drug in clinical circumstances may well produce positive results despite a lack of evidence from placebo-controlled trials. The imperative not to prescribe drugs such that their side-effects outweigh any benefit applies to all our interventions, whether or not a drug has been shown to be effective in a placebo-controlled trial.

Conclusion

To suggest that any and all treatments used in medicine must be assumed to be ineffective unless they have been proved to be better than placebo is to put on one side most of the therapeutic discoveries of the past two millennia. If a new treatment is suggested, it is surely right that it is tested. But let us not assume uncritically that the test *must* be made against placebo. The placebo-controlled trial may provide a gold standard: let us not forget that steel and wood are often more suitable materials to use than gold.

References

1　Jones, B., Jarvis, P., Lewis, J.A. and Ebbutt, A.F. (1996) Trials to assess equivalence: the importance of rigorous methods. *British Medical Journal*, 313: 36–9.
2　Gray, J.A.M. (1997) *Evidence-based Healthcare*. London: Churchill Livingstone.
3　Balair, J., Louis, M., Lavon, P. and Polansky, M. (1984) Studies without internal controls. *New England Journal of Medicine*, 311: 156–63.
4　Hill, A.B. (1963) Medical ethics and controlled trials. *British Medical Journal*, i: 1043–9.
5　Faithfull, S. (1996) How many subjects are needed in a research sample in palliative care? *Palliative Medicine*, 10: 259–61.
6　McQuay, H., Carroll, D. and Moore, A. (1996) Variation in the placebo effect in randomised controlled trials of analgesics: all is as blind as it seems. *Pain*, 64: 331–5.
7　Belison, H. and Friedman, R. (1996) Harnessing the power of the placebo effect and renaming it 'remembered wellness'. *Annual Review of Medicine*, 47: 193–9.
8　McQuay *et al.* (1996) Op. cit.
9　Thalidomide: 20 years on [Editorial] (1981) *Lancet*, 2: 510.
10　Baines, M. and Kirkham, S.R. (1989) Cancer pain, in P.D. Wall and R. Melzack (eds) *Textbook of Pain*, 2nd edition. London: Churchill Livingstone.
11　Thompson, J.W. and Regnard, C. (1995) Pain, in C. Regnard and J.M. Hockley (eds) *Flow Diagrams in Advanced Cancer and Other Diseases*. London: Edward Arnold.

12 Ishister, W.H., Elder, P. and Symons, L. (1990) Non operative management of malignant intestinal obstruction. *Journal of the Royal College of Surgeons of Edinburgh*, 35: 369–72.

13 Baines, M. and Sykes, N. (1993) Gastrointestinal symptoms, in C. Saunders and N. Sykes (eds) *The Management of Terminal Malignant Disease*, 3rd edition. London: Edward Arnold.

14 Schwartz, D., Flamant, R. and Lellouch, J. (1980) *Clinical Trials*, translated by M.J.R. Healy. London: Academic Press.

15 Dunlop, G.M. (1990) A study of the relative frequency and importance of gastrointestinal symptoms and weakness in patients with far-advanced cancer: student paper. *Palliative Medicine*, 4: 37–43.

16 Turner, J.A., Deyo, R.A., Laeser, J.D. *et al.* (1994) The importance of placebo effects in pain treatment and research. *Journal of the American Medical Association*, 271: 1609–14.

17 Belison and Friedman (1996) Op. cit.

18 Elander, G. and Hermeren, G. (1995) Placebo effect and randomised clinical trials. *Theoretical Medicine and Bioethics*, 16 (2): 171–82.

Acknowledgement

Kirkham, S.R. and Abel, J. (1997) Placebo-controlled trials in palliative care: the argument against. *Palliative Medicine*, 11: 489–92.

What is qualitative research and what can it contribute to palliative care?*

DAVID CLARK

Following a rather shaky start, the use of qualitative methods is now gaining increased acceptance within the field of health research. Further progress will have to be made, however, before qualitative research can enjoy the status and respect of other approaches which rely more on techniques of quantification and measurement. It is therefore important to gain a proper understanding of what qualitative methods can contribute to health research, including some agreement on what constitutes rigorous work in this field. Certainly qualitative research seems to hold out a number of possibilities within the area of palliative care. This chapter therefore seeks to map out something of the history, development and content of qualitative methods, while also suggesting ways in which such methods might be used in the service of palliative care research. It will be argued, however, that qualitative research cannot be judged simply as a set of techniques for data collection and analysis. It also comprises a particular way of seeing and a framework for a certain kind of research ethics in which subjective experience is acknowledged and harnessed. Accordingly, it presents researchers with a wide range of practical, political and moral dilemmas – some of which do not arise within other research traditions. Such an argument reveals that, despite lingering claims to the contrary, qualitative methods are no 'soft' option.

Background and development

It is now widely accepted that the particular social, epidemiological and economic conditions of the nineteenth century were instrumental in forging

---

* This is an abridged version of the original paper.

the rise of several new disciplines which turned human subjects into the objects of systematic enquiry. At a time of rapid social change associated with industrialization, urbanization, population growth and technological innovations, the maintenance of social order was seen to depend heavily on knowledge as a form of power. Indeed, knowledge about human subjects could be effective even when other more direct forms of physical control failed. This argument, as developed in the work of the French social philosopher Michel Foucault,[1] is used therefore to explain the rise in the nineteenth century of the new disciplines of sociology, psychology, epidemiology, social statistics and social medicine, all of which were to contribute to social regulation through the accumulation of systematic knowledge and information. Such disciplines were to place a heavy premium on quantification, measurement, and the use of data so derived in the creation of general principles or 'laws' which could be used to explain aspects of society, much in the same way that biology and physics were seeking to explain the natural world. This position we might broadly characterize as one associated with the principles of positivist science.[2]

However, within the human sciences, even by the end of the nineteenth century, counter-claims were to emerge which would challenge this conception of scientific knowledge and offer an alternative framework for enquiry. These claims sought to emphasize questions of meaning, of understanding and of interpretation in making sense of human behaviour and social life. In Germany the distinction was made between the *Naturwissenschaften*, based on the principles of positivism and focused on the natural world, in contrast to the *Geisteswissenschaften*, or human sciences, whose focus was to be more on the meaning of action and the interpretation of the human spirit.[3]

Thus was born the quantitative–qualitative divide. By the early twentieth century some clear schools of qualitative research were beginning to emerge. Outstanding among these was the discipline of anthropology, which began to question its origins as an armchair science and promoted for the first time the notion of 'fieldwork' in alien cultures which would be conducted by anthropologists living in these societies for extended periods, systematically noting and recording what they encountered as 'participant observers'.[4] By the 1920s similar approaches were being adopted by sociologists in Chicago, who were to use the same techniques to study aspects of life in their own city – particularly the worlds of down-and-outs, deviants and those characterized as social 'misfits'.[5] These studies made vivid reading. They had the power to open up the world of others to new audiences; they made claims to authenticity based on a closeness to the subject matter and a willingness to 'get one's hands dirty' in the business of research. By the middle of the century a qualitative research tradition was starting to be identifiable, finding support in such disciplines as sociology, anthropology and criminology. By the 1970s qualitative methods were being explored by researchers in nursing, social work, health promotion and community development. In particular these methods were seen to have something to offer to the burgeoning enterprise of evaluation research, where the goal was some question of practical utility to an organization or group, rather than the elaboration of more theoretical or abstract concerns.[6]

By the late 1980s a substantial body of methodological writing on qualitative research was in evidence. Numerous guides and manuals were appearing and there was an established place for such approaches within the research methodology training of social scientists, nurses and others. The publication of Denzin and Lincoln's *Handbook of Qualitative Research* in 1994 was a landmark.[7] Here was a substantial volume of 643 pages setting out the complete spectrum of the approach, from issues in the philosophy of science, to practical questions of research design and technique. In their introduction, the editors could make the following celebratory claim:

> Where only statistics, experimental designs and survey research once stood, researchers have opened up to ethnography, unstructured interviewing, textual analysis, and historical studies . . . Scholars are now experimenting with the boundaries of interpretation, linking research to social change, delving into the characteristics of race, ethnicity, gender, age, and culture to understand more fully the relationship of the researcher to research.[8]

This quotation reveals two dimensions of the qualitative research approach. The first of these emphasizes the 'toolkit' – the set of skills and techniques which comprise this particular way of working. The second issue is more fundamental and underlies the first; this is the idea of qualitative research as a particular paradigm, with its own theoretical and ideological parameters. Each of these points requires examination in turn, before we can discuss their relevance to palliative care.

The toolkit

The range of techniques which make up the toolkit of qualitative research is now well described in the literature and can be listed as follows:

- observation;
- participant observation;
- interviews (individual, conjoint, group);
- focus groups;
- documentary analysis;
- case studies.

One recent collection contains chapters on each of the key techniques as they apply to health research: observation, interviews, focus groups and case studies.[9] To these should be added also the important area of document-ary analysis. With the exception of the latter, each has now generated an extensive and detailed literature of its own with a good deal of specialist and refined analysis taking place. The purpose here is chiefly to outline the broad spectrum of techniques, by way of overview. For brevity, some associated approaches have been combined into the same passage of discussion.

Observational methods, originating in the anthropological tradition, are sometimes seen as the true essence of qualitative research. Here the researcher will be found at the very heart of the research setting – in the hospital ward, hospice or nursing home, recording in detail naturally occurring events and circumstances. This fieldwork approach will allow the researcher to document conversations, encounters, nonverbal communication, spatial arrangements and the physical environment, all at first hand. These observa-tions will characteristically be constructed as extensive fieldnotes by the researcher, in which are documented the details of particular events, actions, talk and interactions. These are often coupled with the systematic recording, in diary form, of the fieldworker's own professional and personal observa-tions of the research process, including developing insights, hypotheses and theories. Precisely how such observational work is to be conducted can of course often prove problematic. How can a research role be established? How is it explained to the subjects of the study? What ethical problems arise? Are there difficulties in recording items of data without disrupting the study setting itself?

In this sort of study it is rare for the researcher to adopt a purely observa-tional stance in relation to the research setting. For many reasons some form of participation is usual. For example, joining in some of the practical tasks in a hospice day unit, or chatting to patients informally may constitute forms of participation even when the researcher's primary purpose is to observe events without influencing them. It is therefore possible to conceive of a continuum of roles from 'complete observation' through 'observer-as-participant' and 'participant-as-observer' to 'complete participation'.[10] In practice, throughout the course of a study the researcher may adopt all of these on different occasions. What will be important is that in the sub-sequent analysis, the relationship between these different positions and the data collected is classified and made transparent. It is then possible to write an account of the study in which the researcher becomes an active subject within the narrative. At their best such accounts can make compelling and deeply insightful reading. They also present widespread opportunities for validation when the subjects of the research are asked to comment on the inferences and theoretical arguments which the researcher has produced.[11]

Interviewing has perhaps established itself as the most widely adopted technique within the qualitative research toolkit. It is of course a method which can also be used to derive quantitative data, as in the large-scale social survey which seeks answers to a set of carefully predetermined and standardized questions. Qualitative research interviews differ from this in that they are likely to be more interactive in character, with opportunities to develop or deepen the discussion in particular areas, according to the material which arises and the interests and judgement of the researcher. The vehicle for this is usually the *aide memoire*, containing a checklist of key themes or topics which the researcher wishes to cover in the interview. Typically these can be approached in any order, so long as they are all considered and given appropriate attention. In practice such themes may be tackled in a sequential order, for example by encouraging the interviewee to construct a narrative of a particular issue; but the interviewer will also be free to raise topics ahead of schedule, or backtrack if a particular line of enquiry appears fruitful.

It can be seen from this that qualitative research interviews are best conducted by those actively involved in the research process, who will also carry out at least some of the analysis. To be effective, such interviews not only require interactional and communication skills, but also a substantial understanding of the practical or theoretical purpose of the research. In this sense they can be seen to stand at the opposite end of the continuum to, for example, market research or public opinion surveys. Support and supervision is therefore an important component of successful qualitative research practice involving face-to-face techniques. In a context where the interview can at times take on the characteristics of the confessional or counselling encounter, it is important that researchers have a clear understanding of boundaries and tasks and that when the work proves demanding emotionally there are appropriate arrangements in place for debriefing and personal support.[12]

The qualitative research interview can take various forms. Most commonly it is a one-to-one encounter between researcher and interviewee. Sometimes a single researcher may interview two people (e.g. patient and informal carer) or a group of individuals (such as a team of district nurses). On occasions two interviewers may work together. Most qualitative research interviewers and fieldworkers will attempt to frame the researcher encounter as an act of reciprocity. In giving their informed consent, time, experiences and views to a research project, the so-called 'subjects' can reasonably expect something in return. Qualitative researchers will often want to respond to this by showing a willingness, for example, to give additional information about the research, explain their own motivations for doing it or supply further details about relevant local services. This is a large area concerning the ethical conduct of qualitative research[13] and one which acknowledges that the researcher cannot be construed as a neutral, disinterested observer, but must be seen as one with her own values, passions, concerns and preoccupations. Although it is not necessary for such work to turn into autobiography, it is nowadays common for some of these issues to be explored in the published findings of qualitative research.

Individual, conjoint or group interviews have the capacity to generate very large amounts of data. Qualitative researchers will often wish to capture this through tape-recording and subsequent transcription. Such transcripts pose many challenges at the level of analysis and there is now a substantial literature on available approaches.[14] Methods in use can range from simple content analysis, based on the identification of predetermined categories, through the more inductive approaches based on continuous comparison and grounded theory. A number of computer packages are now on the market to assist in sorting and coding items of text, which can facilitate the easy handling of large volumes of such material.

Focus groups involve some of the techniques of qualitative interviewing, but have a rather different design and purpose. They are often used at the early stages of a research project in order to sensitize the researcher to particular themes or issues and they can also be invaluable in allowing a rapid appraisal[15] of viewpoints on a particular matter. In the focus group the researcher will usually act as a facilitator of discussion between a small number of participants, ideally about eight. Sometimes the focus group will share in common some particular characteristic (users of a palliative care service, bereaved carers) or they may be there to represent the interests of a particular locality or professional group; at other times the group will be heterogeneous in character. Usually the facilitator will invite focus group members to discuss a series of topics which has been determined in advance, but the resulting discussion will be steered with a light touch only, in order to promote opportunities for the free-flowing exploration of ideas or experiences. Group processes are seen as an essential element within the technique and must therefore be properly understood by the researcher. Focus groups may have the advantage of encouraging participation in research on the part of those who otherwise feel they have little to say, or those who may be intimidated by a more formal face-to-face interview.[16]

Case studies form a less commonly acknowledged element within the qualitative research toolkit. In truth they are a technique in their own right; a particular approach to structuring research problems and associated design. Case studies can include observation, interviewing and also the analysis of documentary sources. Their attraction to researchers is often the opportunity they afford for triangulation.[17] Using this technique, detailed explication of a single case from a variety of perspectives can allow data drawn from any of the available qualitative methods to be focused on a common issue or research question. Moreover this will be done in ways which allow the particular case to be understood in its wider context. For example, a case study of a single hospice might include the following elements: interviews with individual patients, informal carers, staff and local purchasers; observations of episodes of care in the home, day unit or in-patient area; observation at staff and management meetings; focus groups with volunteers and fund-raisers; documentary analysis of policy and strategic documents, correspondence and minutes of meetings. The aim of such a case study[18] would be to understand the day-to-day work of the hospice and the quality of its service through an analysis of how it relates to other services in the locality, matters of strategic planning, and the views of those who support its work in the wider community. This kind of case study would offer opportunities to triangulate the perspectives of various stakeholders in the organization: health care practitioners, managers, service users, strategic planners, volunteers and fund-raisers. Its benefits would be a more 'holistic' view of the hospice in its wider context.

It may be apparent from this that the methodology of the case study might best be accomplished by a small team of researchers, each with a special interest in specific issues or with particular methodological skills. Case study research using qualitative methods and a team approach provides further opportunities and challenges to develop modes of working which are ethically sound, collaborative and where the involvement of those being 'researched' can be secured at key stages of design, data collection, analysis and dissemination. The case study therefore has the potential to become the exemplar of research as a collaborative or consultative activity involving researchers and those who are the focus of attention in a joint endeavour characterized by mutual respect and shared enthusiasm for new knowledge and insights.

The paradigm

Even from the foregoing, rather cursory description of the 'toolkit' of qualitative methods it will have become apparent that a distinguishing feature of the approach relates to ways of reasoning, modes of perception and styles of asking questions. Jessica Corner[19] has recently explored the Kuhnian notion of 'paradigm' to make sense of research in palliative care. She argues that the current paradigm – that is, a particular combination of theories, applications, modes of measurement – is one heavily dominated by issues of service evaluation and symptom quantification. One inference of her paper is that there has been a dearth of studies which draw on the paradigm associated with qualitative research. This is not a matter of competition or supremacy between approaches, but as Corner implies, we must be aware that qualitative research does have its own starting points and does operate with particular assumptions about the nature of knowledge and understanding. We must recognize in turn that these may not be shared with other orientations based within the paradigm of the natural sciences.

The bases of the qualitative research paradigm are as follows:

- inductive reasoning;
- validity;

- theoretical/purposive sampling;
- 'thick description';
- researcher as interacting subject.

Typically, in such work we would tend to reason inductively, moving from observation to hypothesis, sometimes with only a limited initial understanding of a particular issue and always with a well-developed methodological doubt about the outcome. The qualitative researcher would in turn seek to establish the validity of the data collected, by demonstrating that it has been obtained in ways which tap into the subjects' perceptions, values and meanings. This would be a more important criterion for assessment than concerns with the reliability or replicability of the instrument in use. It would not, however, be an excuse for systematic bias and this should be guarded against and, if necessary, made explicit, where for example some aspect of the researcher's disposition or the chosen method might be seen to have had a specific effect on the data collected and analysed.

Qualitative researchers will be far more willing than others to consider the use of theoretical sampling when identifying subjects. In this approach, samples or study groups are chosen on the basis of the purpose at hand, rather than randomly. This may be particularly appropriate, for example, for case-study research or in-depth observation studies. However, when samples of individuals are being selected there will undoubtedly be some advantages in selecting these from within a known population. A technique known within qualitative research as 'purposive sampling'[20] can be a source of liberation for hard-pressed data gatherers. Within this approach it is considered acceptable to limit the number of subjects in a study to the point where saturation of new information has been achieved. In other words it is not considered necessary (or ethical) to continue gathering data long after it has become clear that nothing new is being learned. This accords with the qualitative researcher's aim to produce what the anthropologist Clifford Geertz called a 'thick description' of the subject matter.[21] In other words the researcher's emphasis will be on sources of variation, nuances of difference, the elicitation of meaning and the understanding of processes, rather than the incidence and prevalence of particular circumstances and events. Finally, as should already be clear, in this paradigm the individual role of the researcher as an interacting subject is acknowledged and the relationship to the object of study is not conceived of as that of the detached observer. Such an approach may involve attending to issues of gender, ethnicity, age or sexuality in the research process, together with their bearing on choice of subject and outcome.

Such a paradigm may appear unfamiliar to those brought up within the traditions of biomedical science. It is important to emphasize, however, that qualitative research is much more than investigative journalism or features writing. There is now a well-developed set of principles for ensuring the appropriate ethical and technical conduct of qualitative research. Within this a strong focus on the adoption of rigorous principles and practices is acknowledged. The intersubjectivity of much qualitative work, especially where it occurs in relation to illness, disease and end-of-life issues, calls for the highest standards of ethical engagement when designing and conducting studies. Good qualitative research has been conducted using opportunistic samples of convenience, but researchers in the field will seek more and more to select samples and study groups in ways which allow them to be located in some wider context or population. Techniques of data collection are now well documented and modes of analysis have developed beyond early, rather individualistic approaches. In short, the best examples of qualitative research currently appearing in the health journals will be seen to follow a set of procedures which is completely recognizable as rigorous and searching in design and execution. As this work becomes more widely disseminated we can look forward to its growing acceptance, adoption and integration within the broader framework of health-related research.

[The section 'Relevance to palliative care' has been omitted at this point].

Prospects and pitfalls

It should by now be clear that qualitative research in palliative care has considerable potential for further development. If this potential is to be realized, however, there must be a continuing emphasis on rigour and the refinement of standards. Some qualitative research has rightly been criticized for a lack of precision, failure to give a proper account of methods of data collection and analysis, and an apparent irrelevance to matters of policy or practice. If these issues can be overcome, then qualitative methods should have a bright future in health-related research in general, and palliative care in particular.

It would be unwise, however, if qualitative research was seen simply as a toolkit to reach the parts that other methods cannot reach. Also important is the wider set of assumptions and practices, the paradigm, which supports it. This key paradigm indicates that the world may not always be as it first appears. Qualitative research has the power to disrupt existing assumptions and to challenge what passes for 'knowledge' in any given context. Opening up to qualitative methods therefore entails a willingness to espouse some of the methodological doubt which goes with them. This does not mean, however, that qualitative research cannot also work in partnership with other methods. Research can be undertaken in which more quantitative work can be used to complement the findings of qualitative data; this is an important point, for qualitative methods should not be seen simply as applicable to the pilot stages which precede the adoption of quantitative research designs.

Qualitative research, however it is undertaken, will only be as good as the questions underpinning it. It should not be seen as an alternative to generating such questions. Of course, by its nature qualitative research is likely to throw up unintended consequences and unexpected findings – it is an approach which allows this to happen. But it cannot be allowed to function as a trawl net, dredging up indiscriminately all which lies in its wake. As the techniques of qualitative research become more refined, so the potential exists to harness these to greater specificity in the setting of research aims and objectives.

Finally, we should keep in mind some of the finer points of qualitative research. Above all this is an approach in which the use of words and the expression of language are at a premium. In appealing for more rigour and methodological accountability, we must remember that pleasure in the written word is also something to be fostered. Poorly written qualitative research can be indigestible fare. Let us therefore look to qualitative researchers for a sense of poetry and a felicity of language which, in building on the insights of the method, create for us a brighter and more perceptive understanding of the world.

References

1 Foucault, M. (1973) *The Birth of the Clinic*. London: Tavistock.
2 Rex, J. (1961) *Key Problems of Sociological Theory*. London: Routledge and Kegan Paul.
3 Giddens, A. (1976) *New Rules of Sociological Method*. London: Hutchinson.
4 Bell, C. and Newby, H. (1971) *Community Studies: An Introduction to the Sociology of the Local Community*. London: Allen & Unwin.
5 Becker, H.S. (1963) *Outsiders*. Glencoe: Free Press.
6 Patton, M.Q. (1990) *Qualitative evaluation and research methods*, 2nd edn. London: Sage.
7 Denzin, N.K. and Lincoln, Y.S. (1994) *Handbook of Qualitative Research*. London: Sage.
8 Ibid.
9 Mays, N. and Pope, C. (eds) (1996) *Qualitative Research in Health Care*. London: BMJ Publishing Group.
10 McCall, G.J. and Simmons, J.L. (1969) *Issues in Participant Observation: A Text and Reader*. Reading, MA: Addison-Wesley.
11 Bloor, M. (1978) On the analysis of observational data: a discussion of the work and uses of inductive techniques and respondent validation. *Sociology*, 12: 545–62.
12 Clark, D. and Haldane, D. (1990) *Wedlocked? Intervention and Research in Marriage*. Cambridge: Polity Press.
13 de Raeve, L. (1994) Ethical issues in palliative care research. *Palliative Medicine*, 8: 298–305.

14 Silverman, D. (1994) *Interpreting Qualitative Data: Methods for Analysing Talk, Text and Interaction*. London: Routledge.
15 Ong, B.N. and Humphris, G. (1994) Rapid appraisal methodologies, in J. Popay and G. Williams (eds) *Researching the People's Health*. London: Routledge.
16 Kitzinger, J. (1996) Introducing focus groups, in N. Mays and C. Pope (eds) *Qualitative Research in Health Care*. London: BMJ Publishing Group.
17 Stake, R.E. (1995) *The Art of Case Study Research*. London: Sage.
18 Ingleton, C., Field, D., Clark, D., Carradice, M. and Crowther, A. (1995) *King's Mill Hospice: Three Years On (1991–94)*, Occasional Paper 16. Sheffield: Trent Palliative Care Centre.
19 Corner, J. (1996) Is there a research paradigm for palliative care? *Palliative Medicine*, 10: 201–8.
20 Strauss, J. and Corbin, J. (1990) *Basics of Qualitative Research: Grounded Theory, Procedures and Techniques*. London: Sage.
21 Geertz, C. (1973) Thick description: toward an interpretative theory of culture, in C. Geertz, *The Interpretation of Cultures*. New York: Basic Books.

Acknowledgement

Clark, D. (1997) What is qualitative research and what can it contribute to palliative care? *Palliative Medicine*, 11: 159–66.

7 Ethical issues in qualitative research in palliative care*

PATRICIA WILKIE

Palliative care involves lessening the severity of an untreatable disease and relieving both physical and psychological symptoms. While palliative care does not involve intensive treatment of the underlying cause of the symptoms some people live for a number of years having regular palliative treatment. Many patients who enter palliative care have already participated in research and may wish to continue to help.

Medical research has two main objectives.[1] These are:

- to increase and refine the body of knowledge on which that part of the practice of medicine which is science-based depends;
- to explore the practical ways in which that knowledge can be applied to the prevention and treatment of disease.

In medical research the primary intention is to advance knowledge so that patients in general may benefit. The individual patient participating in the research may or may not benefit directly from this participation. In medical practice, on the other hand, the intention is to benefit the individual patient and not to gain knowledge of general benefit, though such knowledge may emerge from the clinical experience gained. The distinction between medical research and innovative medical practice derives from the intent.

Researchers always need to adopt the most appropriate research methodology for the subject that they wish to investigate. The qualitative methods of research are appropriate and sympathetic tools for researchers to use when investigating problems in palliative care. Qualitative research most

* This article is a written version of a paper delivered at the Qualitative Research Workshop organized jointly by The Institute of Cancer Research and Marie Curie Cancer Care, held on 11 September 1996 at the Royal Marsden Hospital.

frequently uses the following techniques,[2] all of which are widely used in research:

- in-depth interviews often involving tape recording;
- participant observation, often involving video recording;
- questionnaires;
- focus groups;
- case studies;
- documentary analysis.

Qualitative research is frequently time-consuming and therefore labour-intensive and can be slow. Investigators need to be realistic about the length of time the research will take and about the course of the patient's illness. Investigators often work with smaller samples thus requiring the use of quite sophisticated statistical techniques such as 'Ridits' scales[3] as well as the more common non-parametric tests.[4] The use of smaller samples can make it difficult to persuade researchers accustomed to working with large samples that a piece of palliative research is a rigorous and scientifically valid piece of research.

Declaration of Helsinki

The principles of the World Medical Association Declaration of Helsinki[5] for carrying out research on patients apply to those using qualitative methodologies. The Declaration states that:

- research on human subjects must conform to generally accepted scientific principles and be based on a thorough knowledge of the scientific literature;
- the design of the study should be clearly formulated in an experimental protocol and must be scientifically valid;
- the research should be carried out by scientifically qualified people or supervised by them;
- research should not be carried out unless the importance of the objective is in proportion to the inherent risk to the subject;
- concern for the interests of the subject must always prevail over the interests of science and society;
- each subject must be adequately informed of the aims, methods and potential hazards of the study and the discomfort it may entail, i.e. there must be informed consent;
- in the treatment of a sick person, the physician must be free to use a new diagnostic and therapeutic measure if in his or her judgement it offers hope of saving life, re-establishing health or alleviating suffering;
- in any study every patient should be assured of the best proven diagnostic and therapeutic measures;

• the refusal of a patient to participate must never interfere with the relationship of the doctor with the patient.

Benefits and risks

In research it is necessary to balance the benefits and the risks to the patient. The patient may benefit directly, either immediately or in the future. Much qualitative research in palliative care would be looking at future benefits to patients, so patients participating in the research may themselves not benefit. Most qualitative research would involve minimal or no risk to the patient. But what is a minimal risk? Minimal risk can describe the situation where the level of distress or clinical malaise is slight and where there may be a chance of a reaction which is in itself slight, e.g. a headache or a dry mouth. Alternatively, the risk of such a reaction, if minimal, could be described as less than a person takes driving around the M25 motorway. But, although risks in qualitative research may be difficult to quantify, they may be very real. There may be risks in greater self-knowledge which the person is unable to deal with. There may be a risk of greater understanding of the severity of the patient's situation. The risk of emotional distress or even psychological disturbance as a result of some qualitative research is not understood and needs to be addressed.

Patient consent

Patients need to be informed about the project and what they are being invited to participate in. Before requesting the consent of the patient to participate in the research, the investigator must provide the subject with the following information in a language that is understandable to the patient:[6]

• the aims and methods of the research;
• the expected duration and number of visits to hospital or surgery;
• any foreseeable risks or discomfort the patient may experience as a result of the research;
• the benefits to the patients or others that may reasonably be expected from the research;
• appropriate alternative procedures or courses of treatment;
• that the patient is free to abstain or withdraw at any time.

Deception

Traditionally, there are very few situations where there is an argument for not telling the patient that they are participating in research, e.g. when it would cause distress to reveal the nature of the investigation yet it is in the clinical interest of the patient to participate, or in the case of emergency medicine. But in qualitative research the need for ethically significant deception may arise in psychological research. It may be impossible to study some psychological process without withholding information about the true object of the study or deliberately misleading the participants. According to the British Psychological Society,[7] before conducting such a study the investigators have a special responsibility to:

- determine that alternative procedures avoiding deception or concealment are not available;
- ensure that participants are provided with sufficient information at the earliest stage;
- consult appropriately upon the way that the withholding of information or deliberate deception will be received.

The British Sociological Association (BSA)[8] has similar views. For the BSA, deception of a subject is not permissible in research projects that carry more than minimal risk of harm to the subject. When deception is indispensable to the methods of an experiment the investigators must demonstrate to an ethical review committee that no other research method would suffice, that significant advances could result from the research and that nothing has been withheld that if divulged would cause a reasonable person to refuse to participate. The ethical review committee should determine with the investigator whether and how deceived subjects should be informed of the deception upon completion of the research. The BSA believes that there are serious ethical dangers but that covert methods may avoid certain problems, for example when research participants change their behaviour because they know that they are being studied. It should be remembered that covert methods violate the principles of informed consent and may invade the privacy of those being studied.

Patient participation

It is important for investigators to be aware that patients have varied reasons for participating in a research project. Some patients may very much wish to participate in a project even though their participation may cause them inconvenience, even discomfort, and may also be time-consuming. Patients may wish to help and to 'give'. In addition they may gain from the knowledge that their participation in the research may benefit future patients.

The family may influence the patient's decision whether or not to enter a research project. Some families may wish the patient to participate in research and may encourage the patient to be involved, perhaps because there is a genetic factor in the illness and the information may be useful to the other family members. Some relatives may think that if someone is troubling to involve the patient in research there may still be hope. Conversely, families may be disappointed when their relative agrees to participate, because the time spent in research is precious time which is not being spent with them.

Research is an increasingly important part of both undergraduate and postgraduate education and therefore more staff are becoming involved in research. Some patients may have a particular loyalty to the staff who are carrying out the research and who may also be involved in their day-to-day care and they may not wish to disappoint by declining to participate. Since research also plays an increasingly important part in attracting finance, some patients may fear that if they do not agree to participate they may no longer be looked after by a particular unit or team. If this is indeed the situation it should be discussed with the patient, along with the alternative arrangements for their care in the future. The gaining of consent is very important.

Effect of questionnaires

In any research project the physical, emotional and psychological well-being of research participants must not be adversely affected by research. If the research involves questionnaires, the investigator should have considered the effect of asking questions and of probing into the feelings of the patients. The investigator should be sufficiently skilled to know when to stop asking questions. This highlights the need for rigour in the training and supervision of research staff as well as rigour in research design.

Confidentiality

The confidentiality of the research subject and of the research data must be protected. This is particularly important when the information given in the research may have something to do with the patient's treatment preferences and could involve other staff in the unit. Who is going to know what the patient has said? What is reported to other staff involved in the care of the patient? Investigators need to consider how the confidentiality of the patient will be protected and ensure that the patient is aware of this before joining the project. Storage of data must also be secure.

Recording on tape

Video-recording is often used as a tool in qualitative research. The investigator must be confident that the patient is comfortable with the use of video and understands what will subsequently be done with the tape. Because of the labour-intensive nature of qualitative research, many researchers use audio-recording to record the content of the interview, allowing the interviewer to give his or her full attention to the research subject. Patients must be told of the intention to use audio- and/or video-recording and given the opportunity to refuse. If they refuse they may not then be entered into the study. Researchers may like to consider the possibility of asking patients' consent again at the end of the interview. In this way patients have the benefit of knowing what has been discussed and what has been said. Patients should also be told what happens to the tapes and when they will be destroyed.

Who will have access to data?

Research subjects need to know who will have access to the research data and this needs to be clarified when the patient consents to join the study. Will the patient's general practitioner be informed that the patient is entering a study? Will clinical staff involved in the care of the patient have access to the data? It is possible that some patients may be more willing openly to discuss sensitive and personal issues if they know in advance that the information given is restricted to a very few people.

Intrusion

Social research can be quite intrusive. Subjects are often asked very personal questions in questionnaires. Interviewers often probe into the feelings of the patients. And in focus groups people may find themselves discussing their concerns, their attitudes and their feelings in public. While some patients may find the experience of participating in such research positive, for others the experience may be disturbing. However, the research process may be therapeutic for the patients who believe that for the first time they have been given an opportunity to express their feelings. If participating in the research has become 'therapy' for the patient, what happens when the study finishes? Researchers need to consider such questions.

Even if patients involved in research are not exposed to harm, some research subjects may feel wronged by aspects of the research process. Some patients may perceive apparent intrusions into their private and personal worlds. Some patients may not like discussing with the researcher their relationships with their carers, their partners or their family. Such discussions may make patients feel guilty afterwards.

False hopes

Some research can give rise to false hope. This is a common problem that inexperienced researchers can cause. For example, an undergraduate student wishes to investigate the carers' views of community services for patients with Alzheimer's. In such a piece of work the expectations of the carer for improvements in the services could be raised by the mere fact that the research was being carried out at all. The researcher in this example is unlikely to be able to meet these expectations.

Emotions

Qualitative research often involves working with feelings – feelings about treatments, feelings about pain, feelings about death. Sometimes the patient has coped by not concentrating on certain topics. Investigators need to be sure that they are asking the 'right' questions. Questionnaires need to be clearly thought through and the most appropriate validated questionnaire also needs to be used.[9]

Conclusion

Qualitative research is undoubtedly the best research method for researching many aspects of palliative care. This methodology allows questions about the extent of a problem and the degree of an emotion or feeling to be answered. It is a sensitive method of research when sensitive topics are to be studied. The ethical issues raised in qualitative research are not fundamentally different from the ethical issues facing any other research using patients.

Within the speciality of palliative care much innovative research is undertaken. Research protocols in palliative care must be scientifically and sensitively designed to ensure that patients receiving palliative care are both protected and feel able to participate in the research. Qualitative research can be just as scientifically rigorous as any other methodology and the analysis can be very complex.[10] If researchers are rigorous in their application of sound practice and have carefully addressed the issues discussed in this chapter, ethical problems are lessened. Great vigilance and care is necessary to protect the interests of patients as well as furthering knowledge and benefiting future generations of patients.

References

1 Evans, D. and Evans, M. (1996) *A Decent Proposal: Ethical Review of Clinical Research.* Chichester: John Wiley.

2 Miles, M.B. and Huberman, A.M. (1994) *Qualitative Data Analysis*, 2nd edn. Thousand Oaks, CA: Sage.
3 Agresti, A. (1984) *Analysis of Ordinal Categorical Data*. New York, NY: John Wiley.
4 Robson, C. (1983) *Experiment, Design and Statistics in Psychology*, 2nd edn. Harmondsworth: Penguin.
5 World Medical Association Declaration of Helsinki (1989) *The World Medical Association Handbook of Declarations*.
6 The Royal College of Physicians of London (1996) *Guidelines on the Practice of Ethics Committees in Medical Research Involving Human Subjects*, 3rd edn. London: Royal College of Physicians.
7 Ethical principles for conducting research with human participants (1993) *The Psychologist*, 6 (1).
8 British Sociological Association (1993) *Statement of Ethical Practice*. Annual General Meeting, British Sociological Association.
9 Bowling, A. (1995) *Measuring Disease*. Oxford: Oxford University Press.
10 Miles, M.B. and Huberman, A.M. (1994) Op. cit.

Acknowledgement

Wilkie, P. (1997) Ethical issues in qualitative research in palliative care. *Palliative Medicine*, 11: 321–4.

PART II

Clinical research in palliative care

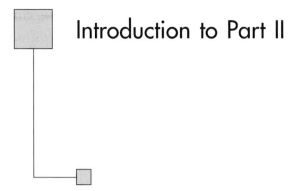

Introduction to Part II

The term 'clinical' has been used to try to capture research that immediately involves people as patients, that attempts to study their particular problems and to evaluate strategies for dealing with these. It excludes the study of services as an entirety, or staff and their concerns. The defining feature of the most useful clinical studies, but paradoxically also the most challenging, are those conducted prospectively, or 'live', as events unfold. These are in contrast to 'after the event' studies such as retrospective studies of case notes, or studies of whole populations, for example those conducted by epidemiologists. There is an immediacy in this kind of research, a desire to understand problems more deeply and to observe carefully how these change or are affected by specific therapeutic strategies, such as in clinical trials of pharmaceutical agents. Encompassed within clinical research is much medical research, but there are many studies conducted by other health professionals too.

The fact that clinical studies are conducted as events unfold, in 'real-time', makes these particularly difficult to conduct, and many issues are yet to be resolved as to how to adapt methods and study designs considered standard in mainstream health care for the palliative care setting. The difficulties are practical, ethical and emotional, and the chapters in this section have been chosen because they illustrate and explore these difficulties. Most of the problems relate to the fact that the people being studied are gravely ill; many may be in the last months, weeks or even days of their lives. Many people working in palliative care have held rather uneasy feelings about research, about the appropriateness of studying people who are at the end of life. In some settings there is a substantial resistance to the idea of research and this is expressed overtly. Elsewhere, the misgivings are less openly expressed but may mean that staff are unwilling to collaborate or cooperate with research; often, and rightly, staff feel very protective of patients and families. Two views exist. One is that research in the palliative care setting places too great a demand on people who are very ill. The other view is that research is an ethical imperative so that quality of care is enhanced. In any event researchers have a duty to consider very carefully the burden they may be imposing on individuals in asking them to participate in a study. There is an absolute requirement to ensure that such studies are carefully designed to reduce burden to a minimum, and to make optimal use of material collected. These data are very precious.

Emotionally, clinical research in palliative care is very demanding. Even practitioners experienced in working in this setting and with the particular client group can find themselves unprepared for the emotional effects orchestrated by studying a problem closely, or by the close and continuous proximity to the ongoing nature of advanced disease. All outcomes of disease and care become known and are closely monitored, in a way that everyday practice does not systematically reveal. In some approaches, such as interviewing, this requires the researcher to hear people's stories and become intimate with these. The close proximity to people's lives while ill or dying, and the emotional impact of this, can be compounded by the isolation and the lack of active clinical input the researcher may have in making the person's predicament better. These together can make researchers emotionally vulnerable. It is wise to establish mechanisms for supervision for the emotional aspect of research; regular contact with an uninvolved person to enable the reseacher to talk over feelings and issues is good practice.

The first chapter in this section is a study of fatigue in advanced cancer by Krishnasamy using a case study method. While this approach is often thought of as qualitative, as in Krishnasamy's study, it also draws data from multiple sources and may involve the use of measurement. Rather like a detective, Krishnasamy sets out to try to understand fatigue and all the factors that may contribute to it, and most importantly to try to understand it from the point of view of the person who is ill. Since fatigue is not well understood, and there are no effective treatments for it, this approach is useful in developing a deep understanding of the problem.

Hinton's authoritative chapter, comparing retrospective reports of terminal illness with those of patients themselves, was selected for inclusion because it sheds light on methods used in prospective and retrospective surveys. As we noted in Part I, surveys of bereaved relatives who are asked to reflect retrospectively on the terminal phase of illness and on care have been used extensively. Yet there has been little work to explore how robust these studies are and how reliably they reflect events reported at the time. Hinton's study casts doubt on the latter and suggests that studies using these methods should be interpreted with caution.

Practically, clinical studies are difficult, as the chapter by Hardy and her colleagues demonstrates. They give an honest and insightful account of their failure to complete a randomized placebo-controlled cross-over trial of dexamethasone for malignant bowel obstruction. The reasons for abandoning the trial are given, along with the sad conclusion that a study of dexamethasone in this context is now unlikely to be undertaken, a salutary lesson for palliative care. Few palliative care services have large numbers of patients relative to the number that may be required to produce statistically meaningful results. This means that a prospective study may have to run for a considerable period of time if sufficient numbers of patients are to be accrued, especially if conducted in a single setting. Indeed, many studies may not be viable in a single setting, and a multicentre study may need to be considered. Eligibility criteria defined for those whom it may be appropriate to approach about participating in a study have the general effect of reducing the pool of patients. The fact that many patients may be too unwell to participate or may be in emotional crisis reduces this pool further. One of the single most important practical challenges for clinical research in palliative care is the ability to recruit a sample of people who are representative of the population of palliative care patients, since there are so many reasons why patients may not be able to participate. The second difficulty is attrition of patients recruited because of disease progression or death; researchers have found various ways of dealing with this problem. Other practical problems relate to selecting appropriate measures for assessing problems or measuring outcomes. Few measures have been specifically designed for the setting, and those that have often have not been thoroughly tested for reliability or validity.

In the next selection, Bredin and her colleagues report on a multicentre study of nursing intervention for breathlessness in lung cancer. Multicentre studies are complex to manage and require very good collaborative relationships as well as the resources to coordinate them. Here the technique of coordinating practitioner-led research from a central research centre, with the support of a clinical trials office and independent data monitoring committee, helped in conducting a complex study. As in most conventional cancer treatment trials there was substantial sample attrition due to illness progression and death, so imputed scores were used for these patients to allow the inclusion of patients with worsening symptoms in the analysis. The steps taken in the management of this study exemplify established 'good practice' in the conduct of clinical trials.

One of the most complex factors that potentially confound clinical research in palliative care is the choice of outcome measures. An outcome measure has been defined as an attributable effect of intervention, or its lack, on a previous state of health. The choice of outcome measure in a clinical study is crucial and has wide-ranging effects on that research, influencing not only the scientific validity and importance of the results but also whether or not they are generalizable. It also affects the feasibility of conducting the research, recruitment and attrition rates as well as patient and researcher satisfaction with the research process. Outcome measures in clinical palliative care research need to be appropriate to the research question, simple enough to be feasible in an ill population of patients, patient-rated (whenever appropriate), ethical, clinically meaningful, validated, sensitive, reliable and repeatable. In addition, they need to be analysable. The chapter by Hearn and Higginson reviews 12 outcome measures that have been used, or have been proposed for use, in the clinical audit of palliative care of patients with advanced cancer, up to 1995. In addition to their use to monitor clinical care, these tools can be used for comparative research, possibly within the context of a social survey. This chapter not only highlights many of the factors which should be considered in selecting appropriate outcome measures for clinical research but also provides an example of the methodology of the systematic review. It should prompt the reader to review critically the use of outcome measures used in other chapters in this book.

Clinical research in palliative care is essential both to demonstrate the effectiveness of current approaches and interventions, and for enhancing quality of care. There is an urgent need to conduct studies so that information can begin to accumulate in sufficient volume to develop the evidence base for palliative care. Solutions need to be found to the practical and methodological challenges in conducting research and this will only be achieved if clinical research is seen as a collaborative and collective effort.

8 Fatigue in advanced cancer: meaning before measurement?*

MEINIR KRISHNASAMY

Background to the study

Fatigue has repeatedly been identified as one of the most common and distressing problems for individuals with cancer[1,2] and the search for a definitive diagnosis for fatigue has resulted in the presentation of numerous hypotheses on the mechanisms involved in its causation.[3] In reality, it is likely that an aspect or aspects of each of the mechanisms postulated play some part in the fatigue experience. There is no universally accepted model of fatigue, but some of the most commonly cited ones which capture various aspects of its multidimensionality, include:

- the Neuromuscular/Central/Peripheral Model;[4]
- the Integrated Fatigue Model;[5]
- Attentional Fatigue;[6]
- the Energy Analysis Model;[7] and
- the Psychobiological-Entropy Model;[8]

Mirroring the complexity of identifying causative factors and establishing cause and effect relationships is an inability to secure a universal definition of fatigue.[9] For example, fatigue has been defined as 'an overwhelming, sustained sense of exhaustion and decreased capacity for physical and mental work'.[10] Following an extensive review of existing literature, analysis of conceptual theories and their own empirical research, Ream and Richardson[11] concluded that 'fatigue is a subjective, unpleasant symptom which incorporates total body feeling ranging from tiredness to exhaustion creating an unrelenting overall condition which interferes with individuals' ability

---

* This paper has been slightly abridged by Meinir Krishnasamy for this publication.

Figure 8.1   Subjective and objective manifestations of fatigue

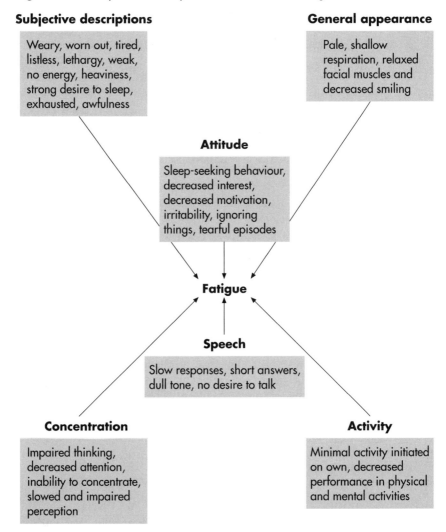

Subjective descriptions

Weary, worn out, tired, listless, lethargy, weak, no energy, heaviness, strong desire to sleep, exhausted, awfulness

General appearance

Pale, shallow respiration, relaxed facial muscles and decreased smiling

Attitude

Sleep-seeking behaviour, decreased interest, decreased motivation, irritability, ignoring things, tearful episodes

Fatigue

Speech

Slow responses, short answers, dull tone, no desire to talk

Concentration

Impaired thinking, decreased attention, inability to concentrate, slowed and impaired perception

Activity

Minimal activity initiated on own, decreased performance in physical and mental activities

to function to their normal capacity' (p. 527). A summary of the subjective and objective manifestations of fatigue drawn from some aspects of the work of numerous authors (Figure 8.1) demonstrates why a universal definition has proved to be so elusive.

As a word, fatigue seems to be unhelpful when used to ask patients to describe their experience of it. A review of the literature demonstrates that people appear instead to complain of a diversity of subjective sensations as outlined in Figure 8.1.[12–19] As a result of this ambiguity, fatigue is often used synonymously with some of the many descriptors presented in

Figure 8.1. However, many of these descriptors have discrete properties which delineate them as concepts in their own right.[20] For example, tiredness has been described as 'a state in which a person feels a temporary lessening of strength and energy',[21] but which may be responsive to self-care initiatives.[22] Lack of energy, general lethargy, exhaustion, lack of motivation, low mood, sleepiness, drowsiness and apathy may all be understood as feelings of fatigue, as well as being recognized as potential causes or consequences of it.[23] These feelings appear to have to be present, although not all at the same time or to the same degree, before an individual can be said to be 'fatigued'. As such, fatigue is understood as a complex phenomenon responsive to, and potentially alternating with, an individual's unique context and experience. For the purpose of this paper, fatigue relates to a subjective, unpleasant, often overwhelming feeling of loss of energy, which interferes with individuals' ability to function to a capacity which they consider to be normal or acceptable.[24,25]

Despite a recognition of its subjective nature, the majority of research undertaken has set out to objectify and quantify the fatigue experience. However, evidence is now emerging from qualitative studies which illustrates the considerable impact of fatigue on individuals' self-esteem, role function, global quality of life, family dynamics, ability to adjust to a diagnosis of cancer, and perceptions of suffering.[26-31] Insights gained from descriptive studies may also prove helpful in the quest to understand better the especially complex relationship between fatigue and depression.[32-34]

To date, attention has focused on the fatigue experienced by patients receiving chemotherapy or radiotherapy, often where recovery is anticipated. Scant attention has been given to the experiences of patients with advanced cancer where the focus of care is directed towards the impact of the disease on the individual and his or her family. In response to a resultant paucity of information, along with philosophical and methodological concerns regarding measurement of poorly understood and defined phenomena, a case study was undertaken to explore the nature and impact of fatigue as experienced by patients, relatives or friends of their choice, and health care professionals involved with their care. Local ethics committee approval was granted prior to undertaking the study.

The method

A case study approach is considered to be germane to the investigation of patient-centred problems[35] as it focuses intensive observation on a single subject.[36] A case study enabled the author to focus on understanding the particular (the fatigue of advanced cancer) in addition to the general (the lived experiences of patients, relatives and professionals) (Figure 8.2). Throughout this case study, the unit of analysis was the experience of

Figure 8.2 The case study design

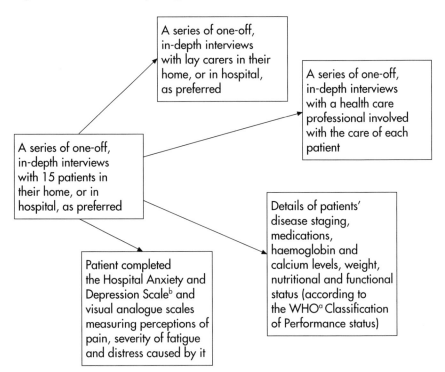

a World Health Organization
b Zigmond, A. and Snaith, R.P. (1983) The Hospital Anxiety and Depression Scale. *Acta Psychiatrica Scandinavica*, 67: 361–70.

fatigue, and a case was defined as incorporating a patient, a relative or friend of their choice, and a health care professional involved with their care. The research design was therefore a multiple case study (where each of the fifteen patients and associated persons represented one case) retaining a single unit of analysis.

As a case study is not restricted by any one methodological consideration[37,38] a triangulation of data sources was included in the study to ensure that objective and subjective data were collected:

- in-depth, tape-recorded, semi-structured interviews;
- a review of medical and nursing case notes, including objective measures of functional status (World Health Organization Performance Status Scale);
- visual analogue scales (VAS) recognized as a valid means of accessing patients' subjective perceptions of the impact of symptoms[39] were used to measure pain (as a factor likely to influence subjective perceptions of fatigue);[40] severity of fatigue; and perception of distress caused by it.[a]

• The Hospital Anxiety and Depression Scales (HADS)[41] was used to screen for psychiatric morbidity in light of an acknowledged, albeit poorly understood, relationship between fatigue, depression and anxiety.[42,b]

Study design: sample

Seven men and eight women, with a variety of cancers, predominantly breast, ovarian, lung and prostate, were interviewed. At the outset of the study a decision to recruit a minimum of 10 patients was based on methodological requirements outlined for studies concerned with gaining insight into individuals' subjective experiences of ill-health.[43] On completion of preliminary analysis following participation by 15 patients, no new information appeared to be emerging from data gathered and a decision to stop recruiting was made at this point.

Patients were recruited from the palliative care unit of a cancer centre in South East England. Patients who described themselves to any member of their health care team as being fatigued/tired/exhausted/etc. were offered letters introducing the study, and were asked to return pre-prepared documentation, stating whether they would be happy to take part. Only patients who had completed their final course of chemotherapy or radiotherapy at least one month previously were eligible to take part. Patients were also asked to nominate a relative or friend and health care professional to be interviewed, so that lay and professional carer perceptions of the impact of fatigue on the patient could also be assessed. Professionals were consequently accessed from a variety of care settings. On receipt of the letters of agreement, contact was made with individuals either in a hospital setting or at their home. In response to participant preferences, seven interviews took place in the patients' homes, while eight occurred in hospital in- and outpatient settings.

Data were gathered from 15 patients, 11 relatives/friends, and 11 health care professionals. Eight patients who had reported feeling fatigued/tired/exhausted etc. and who received letters introducing the study refused to take part. Reasons for declining participation included: feeling too tired (3); already being involved in other studies (3); going away to stay with a relative (1); and finding the topic too distressing (1). Of the four patients who declined to nominate a lay carer, three individuals believed that their fatigue was so intensely subjective that interviewing a relative or friend would offer little insight into the nature of the phenomenon. The fourth individual felt that the study would further intrude upon her already burdened support network. Of the four differing cases where a health care interview did not take place, professionals approached felt they did not know three of the patients well enough to be involved. For each of these three patients, care was or had been provided on an outpatient basis, and two patients had received only minimal contact with the hospital setting.

One patient declined permission to approach a professional involved with her care although permission was given to access her medical and nursing notes.

Following two pilot interviews (not included in the final 15 cases) during which patients spoke with considerable distress of their experiences of living with cancer-related fatigue, a decision was taken to invite patients to complete the VAS and the HADS prior to participation in the interview. It was felt that asking patients to complete the measurement instruments following the interview could have resulted in VAS and HADS scores being affected by individuals' in-depth consideration of their experiences. The WHO scale was completed for each patient by the researcher (MK) following case-note analysis and the interview. Case notes were accessed and data outlined in Figure 8.2 recorded following signed consent to do so by the participants.

Analysis

Data analysis involved categorizing and tabulating data within and across cases.[44] Data were initially considered as fragmented pieces of evidence (e.g. as VAS results or interview themes per individual), before being re-combined and analysed across responder groups (e.g. all patient data or all professional carers' data). Finally data were considered within and across cases, where information from each of the three sources (patient, lay carer and professional) were analysed.

Case note data, performance status scores, VAS and HADS data were subject to descriptive statistics and were categorized and tabulated according to the following headings:

- *Case note data*: Diagnosis and date of diagnosis, date and description of last course of treatment, current medication, medication prescribed within five days of the interview, significant medical events within seven days of the interview (e.g. blood transfusion, increase in pain or breathlessness), significant past medical events (e.g. bereavement, divorce, history of depressive illness), weight, haemoglobin levels, and date of death (where applicable).
- *Fatigue and medications.*
- *Fatigue, infection and antibiotics.*
- *Fatigue and nutrition.*
- *Fatigue anaemia and hypercalcaemia.*
- *Fatigue and performance status.*
- *Performance status and date of death.*
- *Anxiety, depression, pain and fatigue severity.*
- *Anxiety, depression, pain and fatigue distress.*

Findings from these diverse data sources and details necessary to assess the analysis process in depth are presented elsewhere.[45]

Following verbatim transcription, all interviews were subject to processes derived from content analysis[46] and constant comparative method[47] where narratives are searched for supporting and contrasting evidence of key categories and themes. Transcribed data from each participant's interviews were initially coded into micro-categories. Themes arising from this process were then grouped and analysed within and across cases and within responder groups. As the interviews were read and reread micro-categories were refined and key themes were developed. Findings presented below draw on key themes identified from across case comparisons. A single case example is briefly presented to illustrate the way in which data was considered within cases. Although data presented must be considered within the limitations of this study design, insights gained from this case study reflect findings presented elsewhere, where patients experiencing fatigue associated with rheumatoid arthritis, multiple sclerosis and congestive heart failure have been invited to describe its impact on their lives.[48–50]

Key findings from the case study

Fatigue and emotional distress

Fatigue has been described as a classic symptom of anxiety and depression[51] and in several studies of patients with cancer, significant positive correlations between fatigue and depressed mood have been demonstrated.[52–54] The extent to which any relationship between fatigue, anxiety and depression can be considered in responses to the HADS scores in this study is limited, as anticipated at the outset of the project. However, despite the fact that many of the individuals interviewed described their fatigue as being a cause of considerable distress, there was limited evidence of clinical cases of depression (Table 8.1). Furthermore three patients who scored 13, 13 and 15 on the depression subsection of the HADS rejected the suggestion that they might be clinically depressed, believing that their low mood was a normal response to their situation.

The distress caused by the limitations imposed by the fatigue and the advanced nature of their illness is apparent from participants' own words:

> You know, that's what makes me regret, watching myself giving things up, feeling too exhausted to enjoy the people who have given me such pleasure . . .
>
> (Ruth)

For the wife of one man, the watching was very painful:

> I just couldn't stand seeing him like that much longer, it was like watching a candle burn itself out slowly . . . he didn't want to be like

Table 8.1   HADS, WHO performance status, and date of death data

Patient	HADS[a] depression subscale scores	HADS anxiety subscale scores	WHO[b] Rating	Date of death following interview
Margaret	11	9	2	2 months
Edward	13	9	3	
David	9	8	3	7 weeks
April	12	9	3	7 days
Cynthia	10	9	2–3	
Richard	10	7	3	3 weeks
Michael	2	3	1	
Ruth	9	5	2	
Beth	10	12	3–4	2 weeks
Tom	18	3	3	2 weeks
Allan	13	9	1	
Sheila	1	5	1	
Anne	11	7	1	
Gordon	9	6	3	3 months
Enid	15	9	2	

Notes:
a *HADS: Hospital Anxiety and Depression Scale.*[55] Depression ratings of 7 or below were taken to represent non-cases, scores of 8–10 considered doubtful cases, and scores of 11+ were taken to imply definite cases.[56]
b *WHO: World Health Organization Performance Status Scores (range 0–4: where 0 = normal levels of activity and 4 = completely disabled)*

that. I would rather he died now than went on like this for much longer, this isn't Tom, he's gone already.

Throughout the interviews patients described a great sense of loss and sadness at their deteriorating health and limited ability to 'be as they were before':

Sometimes I think, Oh come on Tom make an effort, and then think, No, no, it's no good, I can't for them or me. Fed up, that's it.

(Tom)

To be honest with you, you think you're going mad because you can't shake it off, it just hangs on . . .

(Sheila)

Anxiety did not seem to be a prevalent problem for this group of individuals with only one patient scoring above 10 on the anxiety component of the HADS.

Fatigue and functional status

Functional status represented by World Health Organization (WHO) ratings appeared to offer little insight into the complexity of the fatigue experience (Table 8.1). For each of the patients interviewed, functional ability was described as being highly unpredictable and was thus judged by them to be unhelpful as a means of assessing the impact of the fatigue. Evidence from the case study suggests that fatigue measures currently being completed by patients receiving chemotherapy and radiotherapy may prove to be inappropriate for use with patients with advanced cancer. For example, asking patients with advanced cancer to respond to the statements 'My fatigue is worse in the morning' or 'My fatigue is worse in the afternoon' may prove to be problematic at best, and unreliable at worst, as the very unpredictability of the phenomenon was a major theme throughout the narratives of the patients, relatives and professionals interviewed:

> No I wouldn't say that it's worse at certain times of the day because everything's changed . . . I find that my concentration's gone, everything just gets too much.
>
> (Margaret)

In addition, evidence from the medical and nursing case note analysis suggests that the fatigue of advanced cancer has been locked away, hidden from the consciousness of well-meaning professionals, with very few descriptors of fatigue or interventions intended to minimize its impact recorded in the notes of the patients who took part in the study.

The consequences for patients and their relatives of the obscurity of fatigue became apparent only through the interviews:

> He (a doctor) has no idea . . . he doesn't listen to what it's like, really like to feel like this all the time, you see, they don't take it seriously, this is taking it seriously, talking about it . . . and listening, really listening, to me tell you this is awful.
>
> (Enid)

A case example: Michael, Judith and Claire

Michael, a 53-year-old man diagnosed with mesothelioma in February 1995, had worked as a builder all his life. He lived with his partner Judith and had one 17-year-old daughter. Judith worked as a shop assistant and enjoyed her work and the company and support it offered her, but felt guilty at leaving Michael during the day:

> It's hard to get a balance . . . but you can't just stop it [normal life] . . . but I feel, like . . . he's on his own, what's he thinking?

Box 8.1

Date and description of last course of treatment: Completed a clinical trial seven weeks prior to the interview

Current medication: Occasional Coproxamol; Prednisolone

New medication prescribed within five days of the interview or changes in medication dose: None

Significant medical events within seven days of the interview: None

Significant past medical events prior to cancer diagnosis: None

---

The content of the interviews with Michael and Judith shifted back and forth between the impact of the fatigue and the shock of the diagnosis. For Judith, her sense of Michael's isolation through the loss of social and work roles was the most painful aspect for her at that time. Michael said,

> It drives me mad sitting around here all day doing nothing . . . if it's not being out of breath it's the tiredness . . . I'm used to being busy all day.

He and Judith kept returning throughout their interviews to the impact of the fatigue on his self-esteem and to what they appeared to understand as its significance:

> She'll tell you some days, well, I'm a real, you know very difficult, I get cross and frustrated 'cos I can't help . . . and she gets it, but, well, it has to come out, there's a lot to sort out.

Data from Michael's VAS or HADS disclosed little of this construction of meaning around the fatigue or its significance as a sign that things needed to be 'sorted out'. He scored the distress experienced as a result of the fatigue as 39.7 mm out of a possible 100 mm, and rated its severity at worst as 48 mm out of a possible 100 mm.

Despite describing feelings such as 'I don't want to bother getting up some times, what's the point?', or expressing despondent feelings about the quality of time left to him, Michael scored 2 on the depression subsection of the HADS. When questioned about this low score he said, 'It comes and goes, you have to fight to get on top of it, not to go under.' His WHO score of 1, defined as 'restricted in physical activity but ambulatory and able to carry out light work', did not convey the cost he paid on completion of any 'light work'. Judith said,

> He's just finished when he does anything. The other day he was in the garden, not doing anything heavy you know . . . but he was, well, had to go to bed afterwards.

Box 8.2

HADS score:	Anxiety = 3	Depression = 2
VAS severity of fatigue:	Least fatigued = 9.9 mm	Most fatigued = 48 mm
VAS distress:	39.7 mm	
WHO rating:	1	

Michael said,

> Some days it's so . . . it's . . . I'm just, had enough. I try to do something but either get too short of breath or fall asleep. I can think I don't feel too bad and then by the afternoon I'm used up.

Claire is a staff nurse on a busy general ward at the district general hospital where Michael was first diagnosed. When I approached Michael to take part in the study he had been referred to a specialist cancer centre but it was Claire that both he and Judith identified as the person to speak to for the study. When I asked her why she thought they had been so determined that I should speak with her, she said:

> Oh, I don't know, I think it was because I found out [about the mesothelioma] and didn't shy away from the truth about the inevitable . . . some people need that, but Michael and Judith don't want it . . .

On reviewing Michael's hospital notes there was little evidence of a dialogue having taken place about his fatigue/tiredness/exhaustion etc. and its impact on his life.

When asked who had given him any advice or support regarding this problem he named his wife, a friend who has chronic obstructive airways disease, and Claire. This may be one reason for having referred me to Claire who 'asked me if I was tired and how long for, she, was how can I, um, was expecting me to be tired and warned me' (Michael).

By confining an assessment of the impact of fatigue to the objective measures reported here, its consequences for the quality of remaining life for Michael and his family would have remained hidden.

Box 8.3

Medical descriptors of fatigue in notes: No reference to fatigue/tiredness/exhaustion etc.

Nursing descriptors of fatigue in notes: No documented reports of fatigue

Record of intervention directed at fatigue by professionals: None

---

Discussion

Fatigue, methodology, and palliative care research

Palliative care research should be expected to draw together the physical, psychosocial and emotional components of an individual's experience. And yet, a review of the literature surrounding fatigue suggests a different reality where a reductionist research approach, based almost completely on objectification and measurement, is being applied to a phenomenon of which we have little understanding.

Measurement tools reduce experience to a series of subscales and numerical values,[57] and despite increasing evidence of the limitations of accessing individuals' experiences in this way, we continue to do so – as I have done to some extent in this study. By continuing to approach complex multidimensional phenomena in this way many distressing facets of experience are likely to remain hidden from the clinical and research agenda. Without securing meaning before measurement it is unlikely that an instrument will provide data which can contribute to an understanding of how the phenomenon under investigation impacts on the lives of patients and what factors exacerbate or relieve it.

> I don't think others can feel that sense of loss, just slowly giving up all the things you enjoy; I don't think they can begin to understand that.
>
> (Edward)

Language, meaningful research, and practice development

Descriptors of fatigue used by the patients who took part in this study share a language with that expressed by patients describing chemotherapy- and radiotherapy-induced fatigue, for example, exhaustion, wanting to sleep and lack of energy. By confining an exploration of this phenomenon to objective descriptors or performance status measures designed for patients experiencing radiotherapy- or chemotherapy-induced fatigue, the context of these individuals' experience where meanings are constructed and reconstructed in relation to changing life events is disregarded.[58] For this group of individuals, employing a reductionist approach to the data presented would convey little of the underlying reality, i.e. the progression of the fatigue as it becomes ever more persistent and oppressive:

> I've been tired, but lately it's become an exhaustion.
>
> (April)

> Well now it's got to the state where I just literally want to curl up and stay asleep most of the day.
>
> (Edward)

Exploration of meaning and research with people

The focus of scientific research has been described as the production of objective knowledge about an empirical world, grounded in a belief that inquiry is of value only for what it results in.[59] Within this paradigm, the case study has been described as being of value only because it may generate future research ideas.[60] It could be argued however that without the understanding and insight gained from in-depth exploration, future research for poorly understood phenomena cannot be generated with any degree of certainty. The argument that exploration of meaning in isolation is not definitive is clearly appropriate. However exploration of meaning is no less definitive than experimental research based on inadequately conceptualized multidimensional phenomena.

One question for palliative care research, where the majority of patients who consent to take part do not live to benefit from it, must be whether it can rest comfortably within a research philosophy focused solely on outcomes, to the exclusion of a consideration of patients' experiences of the process of participation. Where exploration of meaning becomes integral to research, the potential for therapeutic benefit and a humanistic research ethic may be maximized.[61] Such an approach, however, challenges us to move away from a tradition that fosters a belief in the unilateral primacy of a scientific research philosophy, and to embrace what has been described as 'much more creativity in method'[62] where previously intractable phenomena such as the fatigue of advanced cancer are no longer reduced to a series of scale values, but are recognized and approached as lived manifestations of advanced cancer.

Conclusion

It is unlikely that fatigue, with its multidimensional composition, will ever be captured fully through reliance on an either/or research approach. As with skilled nursing care a comprehensive and inclusive approach is needed if patients are to benefit and research is to succeed in contributing to practice development. In this instance, a research approach that provided participants with an opportunity to talk about their fatigue was greatly valued by the patients who took part, stating that they felt heard and acknowledged. It would appear that designing research studies that allow patients the opportunity to discuss feelings associated with the intractable problems of advanced cancer will not only provide information necessary to develop professional understanding, but will also contribute to the crucially important work of helping patients 'make sense' of their experiences, not only for themselves, but also for family and friends.

Future developments in the management of the fatigue of advanced cancer do not lie solely with exploration of meaning, However, without an appreciation of the contribution of exploration of meaning to symptom management research, we are in danger of remaining too concerned with aberrant pathology while the fundamental and, to date, largely neglected essence of an individual's lived experience remains hidden, to the detriment of valid research and humanistic inquiry.

Notes

a A VAS is a line of 100 mm in length with anchors at each end to indicate the extremes of a sensation under study. Patients are invited to mark a point along the line that indicates the severity of the sensation currently being experienced. Measuring the millimetres from the low end of the scale to the patient's mark scores the intensity of the sensation. The VAS were included in this study as a means of accessing patients' perceptions of their fatigue in a method substantively different from the interview. The intention was to consider patients' narrative descriptions of their experiences alongside that of a numerical rating, and to compare narrative descriptions of debilitating fatigue (or otherwise) with the VAS scores. The VAS were included to provide a unidimensional, quantifiable, measure of the patients' perception of the severity of their fatigue and the distress caused by it. The intention was not to undertake a comprehensive, quantifiable, measure of fatigue which would have necessitated the use of a multidimensional fatigue assessment instrument.

b The HADS is a 14-item scale developed for use by patients with physical disease. Seven items are concerned with anxiety and seven with depression. A cut off score of 11 is recognized as distinguishing between patients who are coping well with their cancer and those who have developed anxiety or depression.[63]

References

1 Hilfinger, M.D.K., Yeager, K., Dibble, S. and Dodd, M. (1997) Patients' perspectives of fatigue while undergoing chemotherapy. *Oncology Nursing Forum*, 24 (1): 43–8.

2 Loge Havard, J. and Kassa, S. (1998) Fatigue and cancer – prevalence, correlates and measurement. *Progress in Palliative Care*, 6 (2): 43–7.

3 Gall, H. (1996) The basis of cancer fatigue: where does it come from? *European Journal of Cancer Nursing*, 5 (Suppl. 2): 31–4.

4 Gibson, H. and Edwards, R.H.T. (1985) Muscular exercise and fatigue. *Sports Medicine*, 2 (2): 120–32.

5 Piper, B., Lindsay, D. and Dodd, M. (1987) Fatigue mechanisms in cancer patients: developing a nursing theory. *Oncology Nursing Forum*, 14 (6): 17–23.

6 Cimprich, B. (1992) Attentional fatigue following breast cancer surgery. *Research in Nursing and Health*, 15: 199–207.

7 Irvine, D., Vincent, L., Graydon, J., Bubela, N. and Thompson, L. (1994) The prevalence and correlates of fatigue in patients receiving treatment with

chemotherapy and radiotherapy. A comparison with the fatigued experienced by health individuals. *Cancer Nursing*, 17 (5): 367–78.

8 Winningham, M., Nail, L., Burke, M. *et al.* (1994) Fatigue and the cancer experience: the state of the knowledge. *Oncology Nursing Forum*, 21 (1): 23–36.

9 Nail, L. and King, K. (1987) Fatigue. *Seminars in Nursing Oncology*, 3 (4): 257–62.

10 Carpenito, L. (1995) Fatigue, in L. Carpenito (ed.) *Handook of Nursing Diagnosis*, 5th edition. Philadelphia, PA: Lippincott Co.

11 Ream, E. and Richardson, A. (1996) Fatigue: a concept analysis. *International Journal of Nursing Studies*, 33 (5): 519–29.

12 Ibid.

13 Granjean, E. (1970) Fatigue. Its physiological and psychological significance. *The Ergonomics Research Society*, 11 (5): 427–36.

14 Hart, L., Freel, M. and Milde, F. (1990) Fatigue. *Nursing Clinics of North America*, 25 (4): 967–75.

15 Rhoten, D. (1982) Fatigue and the postsurgical patient, in C. Norris (ed.) *Concept Clarification in Nursing*. Rockville, MD: Aspen.

16 Piper, B. (1986) Fatigue, in V.K. Carrieri, A.M. Lindsey and C.W. West (eds) *Pathophysiological Phenomena in Nursing: Human Responses to Illness*. Philadelphia, PA: W.B. Saunders and Co.

17 Glaus, A., Crow, R. and Hammond, S. (1996) A qualitative study to explore the concept of fatigue/tiredness in cancer patients and in healthy individuals. *European Journal of Cancer Care*, 5 (Suppl. 2): 8–23.

18 Krishnasamy, M. (1997) *An Exploration of the Nature and Impact of Fatigue in Advanced Cancer: A Case Study*. London: Macmillan Practice Development Unit, Centre for Cancer and Palliative Care Studies, Institute of Cancer Research.

19 Smets, E., Visser, M., Garssen, B. *et al.* (1998) Understanding the level of fatigue in cancer patients undergoing radiotherapy. *Journal of Psychosomatic Research*, 45 (3): 277–93.

20 Pontempa, K. (1993) Chronic fatigue, in J. Fitzpatrick and J. Stevenson (eds) *Annual Review of Nursing Research*. New York, NY: Springer.

21 Richardson, A. (1995) Fatigue in cancer patients: a review of the literature. *European Journal of Cancer Nursing*, 4 (1): 20–32.

22 Rhodes, V., Watson, P. and Hanson, B. (1988) Patients' descriptions of the influence of tiredness and weakness on self-care abilities. *Cancer Nursing*, 11 (3): 186–94.

23 Walker, L. and Avant, K. (1995) *Strategies for Theory Construction in Nursing*, 3rd edition. London: Appleton Lange.

24 Carpenito, L. (1995) Op. cit.

25 Ream, E. and Richardson, A. (1996) Op. cit.

26 Ibid.

27 Glaus, S. *et al.* (1996) Op. cit.

28 Krishnasamy, M. (1997) Op. cit.

29 Smets, E. *et al.* (1998) Op. cit.

30 Ferrell, B., Grant, M., Dean, G., Funk, B. and Ly, J. (1996) 'Bone tired': the experience of fatigue and its impact on quality of life. *Oncology Nursing Forum*, 23 (10): 1539–47.

31 Vogelzang, N., Breitbart, W., Cella, D. *et al.* (1997) Patient, caregiver and oncologist perceptions of cancer-related fatigue: results of a tripart assessment survey. *Seminars in Haematology*, 34 (3) (Suppl. 2): 4–12.

32 Given, C., Stommel, M., Given, B. *et al.* (1993) The influence of cancer patients' symptoms and functional states on patients' depression and family caregivers' reaction and depression. *Health Psychology*, 12 (4): 277–85.

33 Pawlokioswka, T., Chalder, T., Hirsch, S. *et al.* (1994) Population based study of fatigue and psychological distress. *British Medical Journal*, 308 (19 March): 763–6.

34 Mock, V., Dow Hassey, K., Meares, C. *et al.* (1997) Effects of exercise on fatigue, physical functioning, and emotional distress during radiation therapy for breast cancer. *Oncology Nursing Forum*, 24 (6): 991–1000.

35 Meier, P. and Pugh, E.J. (1986) The case study: a viable approach to clinical research. *Research in Nursing and Health*, 9: 195–202.

36 Yin, R.K. (1994) *Case Study Research. Design and Methods.* London: Sage.

37 Meier, P. and Pugh, E.J. (1986) Op. cit.

38 Yin, R.K. (1994) Op. cit.

39 Gift, A.G. (1989) Visual analogue scales: measurement of subjective phenomena. *Nursing Research*, 38: 286–8.

40 Blesch, K., Paice, J., Wickham, R. *et al.* (1991) Correlates of fatigue in people with lung and breast cancer. *Oncology Nursing Forum*, 18 (1): 81–7.

41 Zigmond, A. and Snaith, R.P. (1983) The Hospital Anxiety and Depression Scale. *Acta Psychiatrica Scandinavica*, 67: 361–70.

42 Given, C. *et al.* (1993) Op. cit.

43 Morse, J. (1994) Designing funded qualitative research, in N. Denzin and Y. Lincoln (eds) *Handbook of Qualitative Research*. London: Sage.

44 Yin, R.K. (1994) Op. cit.

45 Krishnasamy, M. (1997) Op. cit.

46 Morse, J. (1991) Qualitative nursing research: a free for all?, in J. Morse (ed.) *Qualitative Nursing Research: A Contemporary Dialogue*. London: Sage.

47 Glaser, B.G. and Strauss, A.L. (1967) *The Discovery of Grounded Theory.* Chicago, IL: Aldine.

48 Krupp, L., Alvarwz, L., Larocca, N. and Scheinberg, L. (1988) Fatigue in multiple sclerosis. *Archives of Neurology*, 45: 435–7.

49 Crosby, L. (1991) Factors which contribute to fatigue associated with rheumatoid arthritis. *Journal of Advanced Nursing*, 16: 974–81.

50 Schaefer, K. and Potylycki, M. (1993) Fatigue associated with congestive heart failure. Use of Levine's Conservation Model. *Journal of Advanced Nursing*, 18: 260–8.

51 Nail, L. and King, K. (1987) Op. cit.

52 Piper *et al.* (1987) Op. cit.

53 Given, C. *et al.* (1993) Op. cit.

54 Mock, V. *et al.* (1997) Op. cit.

55 Zigmond, A. and Snaith, R.P. (1983) Op. cit.

56 Bowling, A. (1991) *Measuring Health: A Review of Quality of Life Measurement Scales.* Buckingham: Open University Press.

57 Morse, J. (1991) Op. cit.

58 Radley, A. and Billig, M. (1996) Accounts of health and illness: dilemmas and representations. *Sociology of Health and Illness*, 18 (2): 220–40.
59 Reason, P. (1996) Reflections on the purposes of human inquiry. *Qualitative Inquiry*, 2 (1): 15–28.
60 Cassileth, B.R. (1989) Methodologic issues in palliative care psychosocial research. *Journal of Palliative Care*, 5 (4): 5–11.
61 Krishnasamy, M. and Plant, H. (1998) Developing nursing research with people. *International Journal of Nursing Studies*, 35: 79–84.
62 Corner, J. (1996) Is there a research paradigm for palliative care? *Palliative Medicine*, 10: 201–8.
63 Bowling, A. (1991) Op. cit.

Acknowledgement

Reprinted from *International Journal of Nursing Studies*, vol. 5: 401–14, Meinir Krishnasamy, Fatigue in advanced cancer: meaning before measurement? (2000), with permission from Elsevier Science.

How reliable are relatives' retrospective reports of terminal illness? Patients' and relatives' accounts compared*

JOHN HINTON

Introduction

Surveys of terminal illness based on retrospective accounts from relatives have given valuable guidance on people's needs and indicated where care needs improvement.[1] Selecting a representative sample of the population and obtaining retrospective information may be easier than when people are dying, but the lapse of time, the potential influence of relatives' grief and the lack of direct information from patients mean that the data may be inaccurate and biased enough to undermine conclusions. A prospective investigation of patients with terminal cancer[2] included follow-up accounts from the caring relatives to allow comparison of current and retrospective data.

Sample

The sample came from the 428 people with terminal cancer who had been referred to a hospice home care service in two years. The study was intended to assess patients receiving competent care and this unit was chosen for its reputation. These circumstances also minimized avoidable fluctuations in the standard of care and helped to stabilize the assessment results. Of these 428 patients, 69 had no carer at home, 28 were already unconscious or too weak, drowsy or dysphasic to converse adequately, 10 were temporary patients or did not have cancer and 89 died or were admitted within seven days. From the remaining 232, a randomized one in three sample of 77 patients and their relatives were asked if they were willing to

---

* This is an abridged version of the original paper.

be interviewed separately each week about their condition and the help received; nine were replaced by second-choice substitutes because the patient, relative or general practitioner was unwilling. The 43 men and 34 women had a mean age of 65 (SD10), 66 were married, 10 widowed and one single. Their cancers originated in the lung (18), bowel or rectum (11), stomach (11), breast (9) and other sites (28). More details of the participants are available.[3]

Method

Following referral, the patients' and relatives' views were each assessed regularly throughout the terminal illness in semi-structured interviews. The assessments were made weekly for eight weeks, fortnightly for six months and then monthly, usually at home but also when in-patients. All interviews were conducted by the author to maintain consistency. After the death a personal letter was sent to relatives and three months later a visit arranged to make a similar but retrospective assessment.

In each current interview the patient or relative was first asked what problems or troubles had occurred in the last seven days and encouraged, without leading questions, to include them all. Their answers concerning the severity of problems were rated 0 = nil, 1 = discomfort only, 2 = troubling but tolerable, 3 = distressing. Later in each interview a number of selected items were regularly assessed. The declared knowledge of diagnosis was recorded and any statements concerning awareness of dying rated on a 1–9 scale and so was the degree of acceptance of dying if appropriate. The degree of anxiety and the mood for that week were similarly rated and the recipients' opinion of their care (the assessments, with examples, have been described more fully).[4] The time schedule for interviews meant that the minority of patients who lived more than two months after referral had occasional later weeks which were not rated because the current assessments were always for a seven-day period to keep them directly comparable. The follow-up interviews were conducted in a parallel fashion but asking relatives to base their replies upon the whole period following referral to the home care unit, i.e. the period which had been currently assessed.

The relatives' retrospective ratings for this period have been compared with the current ratings. In the comparisons the current ratings were represented by the means of each person's total sequence of weekly ratings, approximated to the nearest whole number. Many calculations have been repeated using the median values. Some final month comparisons have also been made. Agreement between retrospective and prospective data was estimated by Cohen's κ index in the weighted version which gives some credit to partial or near agreement.[5] For most items weightings were applied as for continuous-ordinal rating scales but where scales contained an 'absence' point of greater clinical significance, such as no knowledge of diagnosis or no apparent awareness of dying, a dichotomous-ordinal scale was used as described by Cicchetti.[6] The generally accepted levels of agreement according to κ scores are: 0–0.20 = slight, 0.21–0.40 = fair, 0.41–0.60 = moderate, 0.61–0.80 = substantial and ≥ 0.81 almost perfect agreement.[7] Differences in prevalence given by current and retrospective data (as distinct from disagreement over individual ratings) were estimated by the differences in proportions with 95 per cent confidence intervals (CIs) as for paired samples or by McNemar's test for paired observations. Some results are presented as descriptive categories rather than numerical ratings.

Results

Retrospective assessments of the terminal care period were obtained for 71 of the 77 sample patients (92 per cent). Two relatives had died, one had moved away and three refused. The interviews took place at a median of four months after the patients died, although three were postponed to the ninth month by request. The follow-up assessments were given by the wife (37), husband (22), daughter or daughter-in-law (6), son (3), sister (1), grandson (1) or friend (1). The current assessments of these 71 patients covered a median period of seven weeks, range 1–100. The 570 scheduled current interviews were completed on 566 occasions with relatives and 555 with patients. The last current interview with relatives took place at a median of four days before death, 65 within the final week of the patient's life. The median for patients was slightly longer, five days, because 12 were too weak or insufficiently conscious to describe their state at the last planned interview, although 53 gave adequate accounts even in their last week.

Volunteered symptoms

Table 9.1 first sets out the retrospective ratings of pain against the current ratings by relatives and by patients. For perfect agreement all ratings would lie on the marked diagonals. They clearly do not: for example, six patients who were retrospectively rated 2 (troubled) for pain were not currently reported by relatives to have significant pain and one vice versa. Despite giving some credit to ratings only differing by one, the weighted κ values of 0.11 and 0.12 indicate only slight agreement. In contrast, the patient's and relative's current ratings of pain (Table 9.1, 3rd tabulation) agreed moderately well (κ = 0.52) and showed no gross discrepancies. No pain ratings of 3 (distressing) are shown because this severity was never reached by the mean of current ratings nor given as the overall retrospective rating, although 23 patients had currently reported brief periods of distressing pain and 13 relatives retrospectively described these as atypical episodes.

Table 9.1 Relatives' retrospective ratings of pain compared with patients' and relatives' current ratings, using weighted κ index of agreement

		Retrospective rating				Retrospective rating				Relative's current rating		
		0	1	2		0	1	2		0	1	2
Relative's current rating	0	3	7	6	Patient's current rating · 0	4	5	3	Patient's current rating · 0	9	3	0
	1	6	25	12	1	5	27	17	1	7	36	6
	2	1	5	6	2	1	5	4	2	0	4	6
			κ = 0.11				κ = 0.12				κ = 0.52**	

Pain ratings: 0 = nil, 1 = discomfort, 2 = troubling but tolerable.
** Moderate agreement.

These calculations have been repeated using the current median values in case the means did not adequately represent the overall degree of pain, but the agreement levels hardly changed; the κ values for the retrospective/current comparisons were 0.14 for patients and 0.12 for relatives but 0.54 between the two current ratings.

Pain was generally rated more severe retrospectively, a bias indicated by the distribution of more ratings above the diagonals in Table 9.1. At the follow-up 34 per cent were rated 2 (troubled) compared with 14 per cent in patients' current reports (difference 20 per cent, CI 6–33 per cent) and 17 per cent in the relatives' (difference 17 per cent, CI 4–30 per cent). Current pain ratings from relatives compared with patients, however, showed no clear bias.

The retrospective and current ratings of the other commonly volunteered problems have been similarly compared and the levels of agreement are given in Table 9.2 (in the order of symptom frequency given at follow-up). The reports of pain and appetite loss appear least reliable. Relatives were also inconsistent about patients' anxiety, rating five patients as 'troubled' at follow-up whom they had not currently reported as anxious. Three of these five patients had in fact volunteered their own anxiety, so that for this symptom the relatives' retrospective accounts moved towards the patients'. Some other symptom reports proved more reliable. Immobility ratings showed substantial agreement between retrospective and current accounts with the κ values of 0.68 and 0.66, while dyspnoea (breathlessness), nausea/vomiting and the relatives' ratings of confusion showed moderate agreement.

Agreement between retrospective and current ratings for any problem was always worse than that between the two current reports, as Table 9.2

Table 9.2   Levels of agreement between ratings of problems volunteered at follow-up and current ratings from patients and relatives estimated by weighted κ index (*n* = 71)

Problem	Retrospective cf. relative's current rating κ	Retrospective cf. patient's current rating κ	Relative's current cf. patient's current rating κ
Patients' symptoms			
Pain	0.11	0.12	0.52**
Weakness	0.25*	0.21*	0.75***
Vomiting/nausea	0.43**	0.36*	0.70***
Dyspnoea	0.54**	0.54**	0.85****
Constipation	0.25*	0.28*	0.77***
Confusion	0.50**	0.13	0.32*
Depression	0.21*	0.16	0.53**
Anxiety	0.04	0.43**	0.65***
Immobility	0.68***	0.66***	0.93****
Anorexia	0.03	0.09	0.35*
Malaise/fever	0.14	0.29*	0.56**
Relatives' symptoms			
Strain of caring	0.22*	−0.06	0.23*
Relative ill	0.36*	0.12	0.52**

Agreement: *fair. **moderate. ***substantial. ****almost perfect.

shows (except for patients with mental confusion). Current accounts of reduced mobility and dyspnoea from patients and relatives agreed almost perfectly and several other symptoms showed substantial agreement. In case agreement between the two current ratings appeared greater because the means from several interviews were compared, κ scores were also calculated for some single week ratings, but this only made the two current accounts agree more closely. Kappa indices for the first week, for example, were 0.60 for pain, 0.81 for weakness and 0.80 for nausea/vomiting and results for the second week were similar, all higher than the Table 9.2 figures. They further emphasized the reduction in reliability of reports during the interval between current and retrospective assessments.

[We have omitted more detailed analysis at this point. Eds.]

The period prevalences of some common problems as volunteered retrospectively and currently have been compared for possible bias. All symptoms were less often rated 'discomfort only' at the follow-up. This difference reached statistical significance for the patients' reports of pain (difference 15 per cent, CI 2–32 per cent), for current reports of weakness by relatives

Table 9.3 Relatives' retrospective account of patients' recognition of terminal cancer and their mood compared with current assessments directly from patient

Assessment	Retrospective rating (%)	Mean current rating (%)	κ
Diagnosis			
Known	62 (87)	63 (89)	0.70***
Partly known	5 (7)	5 (7)	
Not known	4 (6)	3 (4)	
Awareness of dying			
Certain	40 (56)	29 (41)	0.50**
Probable	10 (14)	16 (23)	
Possible	12 (17)	19 (27)	
Not acknowledged	9 (13)	7 (10)	
Acceptance of dying			
Full	16 (27)	6 (10)	0.41**
Nearly full	19 (32)	16 (27)	
Some	21 (35)	33 (55)	
Nil	4 (7)	5 (8)	
Mood			
Cheerful	23 (32)	15 (21)	0.19
Equable	35 (49)	34 (48)	
Sad/depressed	13 (18)	22 (31)	
Anxiety			
Calm	29 (41)	24 (34)	0.41**
Normal concern	27 (38)	31 (44)	
Worried/anxious	15 (21)	16 (23)	

Weighted κ index: **moderate. ***substantial agreement.

(difference 24 per cent, CI 10–38 per cent) or by patients (difference 17 per cent, CI 2–30 per cent), and for patients' reports of nausea and/or vomiting (difference 14 per cent, CI 2–27 per cent). The retrospective ratings of 'discomfort only' for the other symptoms were given to fewer than the 10 per cent necessary for comparison of percentage by this formula.

[We have omitted Hinton's more detailed analysis here. He reports that in addition to this general tendency for relatives not to describe symptoms retrospectively as 'discomfort only', there was a bias in one or other direction for certain symptoms. Although pain tended to be rated as more intense retrospectively, patients' weakness, depression, and malaise and the relatives' own sense of strain were reported significantly less frequently at the follow-up interview than in the current accounts. Eds.]

Table 9.4   Current and retrospective assessments of relatives' mood and fatigue

Assessment	Retrospective rating (%)	Mean current rating (%)	κ
Relative's mood			
Cheerful	12 (17)	9 (13)	0.25*
Equable	40 (56)	41 (58)	
Sad/depressed	19 (27)	21 (30)	
Relative's anxiety			
Calm	16 (23)	9 (13)	0.33*
Normal concern	35 (49)	39 (55)	
Worried/anxious	20 (28)	23 (32)	
Relative's fatigue			
Nil	16 (23)	9 (13)	0.40**
Some fatigue	35 (49)	39 (55)	
Very tired/exhausted	20 (28)	23 (32)	

Weighted κ index: *fair agreement. **moderate agreement.

Regular assessments of patients' and relatives' reactions

The mean ratings from the assessments of each patient's knowledge and attitude towards his or her illness have been assigned to the categories shown in Table 9.3. The current assessments showed that nearly 90 per cent of patients knew they had a type of cancer, which substantially agreed with relatives' retrospective assessments. The follow-up ratings of patients' awareness of dying agreed moderately well with the direct assessments, although relatives considered 56 per cent were certain they were dying, 15 per cent higher (CI 3–28 per cent) than the current figure. The retrospective ratings of patients' acceptance of dying also agreed moderately well with current assessments, although relatives again recalled a higher proportion as fully accepting death (difference 17 per cent, CI 7–26 per cent).

Relatives' retrospective estimates of patients' mood were less reliable, showing only slight agreement with current assessments (see Table 9.3). Fewer patients were retrospectively considered sad or depressed compared with the regular direct patient assessments (difference 13 per cent, CI 0–25 per cent). This bias is similar to the retrospective underestimate of depression when volunteered as a symptom. The follow-up assessments of the degree of patients' anxiety or calmness were rather better, showing moderate agreement with patients' self-description. The relatives' current and retrospective assessment of their own earlier emotional state (see Table 9.4) showed fairly similar agreement levels to their reports on patients' feelings. Relatives did not retrospectively underrate their own earlier depression, however, and four spontaneously remarked at the follow-up that their grief had reached distressing levels during the care period. Other regular assessments of the relatives' state included their fatigue, which showed moderate agreement.

The relatives' current opinion of care was excellent or very good in 59 per cent, good in 38 per cent and 3 per cent were just satisfied. None expressed general dissatisfaction. At follow-up relatives increased their praise with 72 per cent in the very positive group (difference 13 per cent, CI 1–24 per cent). Despite this later positive bias, the relatives' retrospective and current opinions agreed moderately well ($\kappa = 0.42$). The relatives' retrospective opinions showed a lesser degree of agreement with the individual patients' ratings ($\kappa = 0.24$) although, as groups, the distributions of their current opinion of care had been very similar.

The last month

As some qualities studied could change as patients came closer to dying, comparisons were repeated using later interviews only. During the last month a median of three interviews were completed with the 71 patients and with the relatives; all completed at least one. Retrospective reports of troubling symptoms did not generally agree more closely with current reports by selecting only those in the last month, although small changes occurred. For most symptoms κ indices kept within 0.10 of their values for the whole period. Six symptoms gave higher mean current ratings during the last month and in five the κ indices changed by 0.10–0.20. Agreement worsened slightly for patients' reports of malaise ($\kappa = 0.18$) and for relatives' reports of weakness ($\kappa = 0.12$) and confusion ($\kappa = 0.36$) and improved slightly for symptom reports of anxiety by patients and relatives ($\kappa = 0.63$ and 0.18) and for patients' reports of pain ($\kappa = 0.26$).

In the regular assessments the average proportion of patients currently considered to be certain that they were dying was 41 per cent according to means for the whole period, 44 per cent for the last month and it was 46 per cent in the last assessment only. The κ indices of agreement with relatives' follow-up ratings of patients' awareness were 0.50, 0.57 and 0.60 respectively, not so very different. Full or nearly full acceptance of dying was found in 37 per cent for the whole period, 51 per cent for the last month and 53 per cent for the last interview compared with the 58 per cent given by relatives retrospectively. The κ values were 0.41, 0.46 and 0.42 respectively. It appears that the reliability of individual ratings of these attitudes improved little by focusing on later current interviews, although the distribution of retrospective ratings of acceptance more closely resembled the patients' final state. The means of the regular assessments of patients' anxiety during the last month showed similar agreement with the retrospective ratings as the means for the whole period ($\kappa = 0.41$ and 0.47 respectively). The last month's ratings of patients being sad or depressed, however, matched the follow-up report at no better than chance level ($\kappa = 0.02$); 42 per cent of patients currently described a lowered mood compared with the relatives' retrospective estimate of only 18 per cent (difference 24 per cent, CI 10–38 per cent).

Discussion

The apparent unreliability of several aspects of relatives' retrospective accounts of terminal illness is disappointing, but this study itself needs critical evaluation and comparison with the other sparse evidence available before reaching that conclusion.

This sample was not truly representative of the population, and generalizations from its results need caution. In practice it is virtually impossible to obtain current, repeated, detailed assessments throughout the terminal illness of a fully randomized group; prospective studies are more limited than retrospective surveys in their population samples by difficulties in obtaining the necessary willing cooperation of many people in the time available and by ethical restraints. These patients were a random sample from only one district service although they did not appear any more atypical than any other such samples. They acted as their own controls in statistical comparisons and only the differences or agreement between current and retrospective reports have been considered here, so that selection bias should only affect the broad conclusions if this group were extraordinarily unreliable.

Subjective data are by nature imprecise and techniques of measurement may influence results by their manner of presentation or the inevitable interaction between subject and assessor. The open-ended interview technique is particularly vulnerable to bias but, despite the acknowledged weaknesses of the method chosen,[8] it made it possible to continue assessments as patients neared death and avoided the influence of predetermined selective questions. The softness of this data was partly offset by comparing data from the same subjects by the same assessor. Not using checklists might increase omissions but the risk was accepted as part of the price of allowing patients and relatives to choose what they thought relevant. The open-ended technique could be checked against regular assessments in two items, depression and anxiety. Even though spontaneous reports of these symptoms sometimes differed from the regular assessment ratings at the same interview, the levels of agreement between patients' current and relatives' retrospective accounts proved very similar by either method, slight agreement for depression ($\kappa = 0.16$ and 0.19) and moderate agreement ($\kappa = 0.43$ and 0.41) for anxiety. Evidently the method of assessment did not account for the differences between current and follow-up ratings.

The variable duration of assessment periods in this study could possibly affect the results. Other enquiries have chosen the last year, eight or four weeks before death, the 'terminal illness' or just one opportune interview. In this prospective study where death was expected but not accurately predictable, there appeared no reason to consider any remaining period less or more important, so all the time from referral until death was assessed and relatives asked to evaluate the same retrospectively. In fact, the levels of agreement between follow-up and most current ratings were very similar in these patients whether all current interviews or just those in the final month were considered. Where mean ratings had altered in the last month the κ scores rose a little for two items and fell in three. Therefore, in this study the reliability of individual ratings was not greatly affected by the period chosen, although some group distributions of ratings became slightly closer or further from the distributions given at follow-up.

Lastly, the means of current ratings were only approximate measures of the whole care period. Means can hide brief isolated episodes of suffering although, in compensation, they avoid over-emphasizing one fluctuation in a usually tolerable condition. Interviewing provided many reminders that a numerical rating, although useful, can be an astringent over-simplification of people's experience, either for a single week or the whole terminal period. Evaluating people's perception of a dying relative by accuracy alone is, after all, a very narrow judgement. Other arithmetic measures were tried. Medians of all current ratings agreed with the follow-up at similar levels to means. Medians of positive ratings only, which ignored symptom-free weeks and emphasized any severe episodes, gave higher current scores and made agreement with retrospective ratings worse for most symptoms. The exceptions were the relatives' reports of patients' pain or anxiety symptoms. Perhaps episodes of these particular symptoms more often leave lasting impressions which affect retrospective views.

If, despite its imperfections, this study is considered a good enough comparison of current assessments and relatives' retrospective accounts, the conclusion is that relatives' retrospective reports of certain important symptoms cannot be relied on. Their current reports agreed much better with what patients were describing. In particular, the retrospective estimates of pain severity agreed poorly with what patients and relatives had stated at the time and became biased towards greater severity. This warns that when evaluating care, retrospective pain descriptions could well mislead. Weakness and depression were significantly underestimated at the follow-up. In general, symptoms were less likely to be described as 'discomfort only' at the follow-up and more likely to be recalled as 'troubling' or omitted altogether.

Many items in relatives' retrospective accounts, however, did agree moderately well with current descriptions, for example, symptoms of dyspnoea, vomiting and reduced mobility. Their retrospective view of patients' knowledge of the diagnosis was substantially correct. Relatives' recall of patients' awareness and acceptance of dying agreed moderately well with direct assessments from patients although they favoured memories of patients' final level of acceptance. The relatives' follow-up reports of patients' anxiety accorded moderately well with the patients' own comments and with the regular current assessments (but not with what the relatives had volunteered about the patients at the time). Retrospective assessments of the relatives' own mood, anxiety and fatigue were in fair to moderate agreement with the regular current assessments.

These results are quite compatible with the few other comparisons available, although assessments and statistical techniques differ. Ahmedzai et al.[9] found that ratings of pain, constipation and appetite by 40 patients with lung cancer in the last month of life did not correlate significantly (0.24–0.26) with relatives' reports 6–24 months after the death but reached 0.56 for dyspnoea (correlation coefficients are generally higher than κ scores). They also found retrospective scores for being sad/miserable were less than the current scores while mean scores for frightened/panic stayed equal; the correlations were only 0.36 and 0.22 respectively (not significant). The relatives' estimate of patients' awareness of dying were slightly higher than patients' statements to staff but did not differ significantly. Cartwright and Seale[10] tested the validity of their own survey method by comparing retrospective interviews of relatives with an available assessment from 34 patients made 1–21 weeks before the death. They found poor congruence (mean squared contingency) between the two assessments regarding 14 symptoms 'in the last twelve months', except for constipation, and 'not high' between relatives' retrospective and patients' current opinion of care. Higginson et al.[11] compared relatives' retrospective ratings of 'the last week of the patient's life' with available interviews of six patients and seven family members within the final three weeks and found poor agreement for pain and for anxiety in patients and relatives. They also noted that retrospective ratings of symptoms tended to polarize.

The evidence of inconsistencies does not mean that retrospective reports should be dismissed. Many relatives in the present series gave accurate follow-up accounts or recounted events in detail. They usually differentiated isolated acute episodes of distress from the overall level of comfort. Some did include such conflicting or bland statements as to invite understanding more than belief. Faults did not lie entirely with the retrospective accounts; for instance the follow-up ratings of one symptom, anxiety, veered more towards the patients' viewpoint than relatives' own current reports: hindsight has some benefits. Nevertheless, the two current reports consistently agreed better with each other than either did with the follow-up which does make the retrospective data more suspect.

Conclusion

The accuracy of retrospective reports is well conveyed by the curate's response to the bishop's comment on his doubtful egg in the classic *Punch* cartoon of just 100 years ago.[12] 'Oh no, my lord, I assure you! Parts of it are excellent.' Retrospective reports of terminal illness from relatives require cautious interpretation and plans for such surveys should now consider selecting the more reliable items. For estimates of certain symptoms such as pain, weakness or depression, current assessments are far preferable.

References

1 Cartwright, A., Hockey, L. and Anderson, J. (1973) *Life Before Death*. London: Routledge and Kegan Paul.

2 Hinton, J. (1994) Can home care maintain an acceptable quality of life for patients with terminal cancer and their relatives? *Palliative Medicine*, 8: 183.

3 Ibid.

4 Ibid.

5 Cohen, J. (1960) A coefficient of agreement for nominal scales. *Educational and Psychological Measurement*, 20: 37.

6 Cicchetti, D.V. (1976) Assessing inter-rater reliability for rating scales: resolving some basic issues. *British Journal of Psychiatry*, 129: 452.

7 Landis, J.R. and Koch, G.G. (1977) The measurement of observer agreement for categorical data. *Biometrics*, 33: 159.

8 Ahmedzai, S., Morton, A., Reid, J.T. and Stevenson, R.D. (1988) Quality of death from lung cancer: patients' reports and relatives' retrospective opinions, in M. Watson, S. Greer and C. Thomas (eds) *Psychosocial Oncology*. Oxford: Pergamon.

9 Ibid.

10 Cartwright, A. and Seale, C. (1990) *The Natural History of a Survey: An Account of the Methodological Issues Encountered in a Study of Life Before Death*. London: King Edward's Hospital Fund.

11 Higginson, I., Priest, P. and McCarthy, M. (1994) Are bereaved family members a valid proxy for a patient's assessment of dying? *Social Science and Medicine*, 38: 553.

12 *Punch*, 109: 222, 1895.

Acknowledgements

I am very grateful to these patients and relatives who gave such willing help. The study was supported by a Department of Health grant.

Reprinted from Hinton, John (1996) 'How reliable are relatives' retrospective reports of terminal illness? Patients' and relatives' accounts compared', *Social Science and Medicine*, 43 (8): 1229–36. With permission from Elsevier Science.

10 Pitfalls in placebo-controlled trials in palliative care: dexamethasone for the palliation of malignant bowel obstruction

JANET R. HARDY, JULIE LING,
JANINE MANSI, RICHARD ISAACS,
JUDITH BLISS, ROGER A'HERN,
PETER BLAKE, MARTIN GORE,
JOHN SHEPHERD AND GEOFF HANKS

Introduction

Bowel obstruction is not an uncommon problem in advanced malignant disease, especially in ovarian cancer. Occasionally, surgery can result in useful palliation, but this is not always possible or appropriate in this patient group. To date, traditional conservative medical management has consisted of intravenous fluids, nasogastric suction, analgesia and anti-emetics.[1-4]

Dexamethasone has been used in some centres to palliate the symptoms of obstruction, and to attempt to speed up its resolution.[5-7] It is thought that the anti-inflammatory activity of steroids may reduce the swelling associated with a malignant lesion and thus relieve obstruction.[8] The side-effects of dexamethasone are well documented. The short-term toxicities include gastric irritation, oral candidiasis, agitation and exacerbation of pre-existing diabetes. More long-term complications include proximal weakness and the development of a cushingoid habitus.[9]

In an attempt to confirm a benefit in bowel obstruction, two randomized placebo-controlled trials of dexamethasone versus normal saline in patients with bowel obstruction have been undertaken in this hospital (Royal Marsden, London). These studies illustrate the course and outcome of bowel obstruction in the context of malignant disease, and the difficulty in conducting placebo-controlled studies of what is considered a standard treatment, even where there has been no proven benefit of such a treatment.

Materials and methods

This was designed as a double-blind, placebo-controlled crossover study.

Eligible patients were those with a histological diagnosis of carcinoma, advanced intra-abdominal disease and symptoms (including vomiting, abdominal distension, abdominal colic, constipation) and signs (distended abdomen, obstructive bowel sounds) of obstruction plus radiological evidence of obstruction (such as altered fluid levels, dilated bowel or absent gas in large bowel). Patients with a history of gastrointestinal haemorrhage, active peptic ulceration, a previous adverse reaction to steroids, signs of peritonism or those who were already on intravenous fluids or steroids were excluded.

Patients were stratified into two groups, 'on treatment' and 'off treatment', according to whether or not they had received any specific systemic anti-cancer therapy (in the form of chemotherapy) within the previous 28 days. Patients on palliative hormonal therapy were not considered as being 'on treatment'.

Following written informed consent, patients were randomized to receive either placebo (normal saline) or dexamethasone 4 mg intravenously (iv), every six hours for five days. If the obstruction resolved (as defined below), iv therapy was discontinued. If the obstruction was still present at Day 5, the patient was 'crossed over' to the other arm of the study for a further five days. Syringes were labelled Days 1–5 and Days 6–10, so that treatment was blind to all but the pharmacy staff. The study was terminated on Day 10 with further treatment given as thought appropriate by the attending physician.

All patients received standardized medical management as shown in Figure 10.1. A surgical team was notified of all cases. Patients were assessed daily to monitor fluid intake, bowel activity, episodes of vomiting, as well as analgesic and anti-emetic requirements. Toxicity was documented as the worst episode of any symptom during the preceding 24 hours on a four-point scale (none, mild, moderate, severe).

The primary end-point of the study was outcome at Day 5. Secondary end-points included outcome at Day 10, side-effects of 'treatment' and survival.

Response was defined as the resolution of the bowel obstruction at Day 5, as evidenced by the absence of vomiting, the ability to tolerate a light diet and the presence of bowel flatus or movement.

An initial trial was terminated following the departure of the primary investigator (Trial 1). The study was subsequently reopened with minor modifications in an attempt to improve patient accrual. Trial 2 allowed any patient with symptoms or signs of bowel obstruction (confirmed radiologically) and those patients already on intravenous fluids, as long as they had not been in established obstruction for more than 12 hours. It also allowed for patients with previous episodes of obstruction.

Figure 10.1   Medical management of bowel obstruction

Fluid balance

Intravenous (iv) fluids to be given 1 l, every 8 h initially, and then as per fluid balance (saline or 5% dextrose according to electrolytes).

Nasogastric tube on free drainage, if possible and/or appropriate.

Oral fluids:

- initially clear fluids ≤ 10 ml hourly;
- if no vomiting for 24 hours increase to 30 ml hourly;
- if no vomiting for 24 hours increase to 60 ml hourly;
- then free fluids for 24 hours;
- then low residue diet (refer to dietitian);
- if vomiting occurs at any of the above stages, to return to previous stage for a further 24 hours.

Analgesia

For colic or general abdominal pain, start with Buscopan 20 mg *per os*/iv as required to be taken four times a day ± mebeverine 135 mg to be taken three times a day *per os* if tolerated.

If opioids are required, use diamorphine in subcutaneous infusion.

If dyspepsia is a problem, iv cimetidine 200 mg to be taken three times a day and mucaine 10 ml to be taken four times a day *per os* or via nasogastric tube if tolerated.

Anti-emetics

Haloperidol 3 mg per day in subcutaneous infusion or 1.5 mg *per os* twice a day if tolerated. If no response, add cyclizine suppositories.

Laxatives

Suppositories (glycerine) if faeces on rectal examination on day 1, then as indicated.

Aperients (softeners only, e.g. Milpar 10 ml twice a day *per os* or docusate 100 mg twice a day *per os*) if tolerated from Day 1.

Results

Trial 1 was commenced in December 1987. Accrual to this study was slow and only 25 patients were recruited over a 36-month period. The study was reopened in January 1993 (Trial 2). Recruitment was again slow (14 patients in 24 months) and the study was finally terminated after 24 months, when only 14 patients had been recruited and it appeared no longer viable.

Table 10.1   Patient characteristics

	Trial 1	Trial 2	Combined
Randomized	25	14	39
Commenced study	23	14	37
Age			
median (years)	57	59	59
range	(44–80)	(38–65)	(38–80)
Previous and/or current chemotherapy	20/23	14/14	34/37
Time from diagnosis to obstruction			
median (months)	11	18	13
range	(1–120+)	(1–85)	(1–120+)
Time from obstruction to death			
median (months)	2	4.5	2.5
range	(<1–18.5)	(1–18)	(<1–18.5)
Time from diagnosis to death			
median (months)	15	19.5	19
range	(2–120+)	(7–98)	(2–120+)

Patient characteristics are shown in Table 10.1. All patients were female and the majority had a diagnosis of ovarian cancer. Their median age was 59 years (range 38–80). The majority of patients had previously been treated with one or more courses of chemotherapy prior to the development of their bowel obstruction.

Across all patients, the median time from diagnosis of the malignancy to the development of obstruction was 13 months (range 1–120+ months). The median time from obstruction to death was 2.5 months (range < 1–18.5 months) and the median overall survival (diagnosis to death) was 19 months (range 2–120+ months).

Trial 1

Twenty-five patients were randomized in this study, but two patients withdrew prior to the start. Of those that commenced the study, 13 patients were randomized to receive dexamethasone and 10 received placebo (see Table 10.2).

Thirteen of the 23 patients were classed as 'on treatment' (chemotherapy within 28 days of study). In 11 of these patients, there was resolution of the obstruction by Day 5 (eight out of eight patients who had been randomized

Table 10.2 Response

	Trial 1	Trial 2	Combined
Overall response rate	15/22	6/13	21/35 (60%)
Response in points on treatment[a]	11/13	3/7	14/20 (70%)
Response in points not on treatment	4/9	3/6	7/15 (47%)
Response in points on treatment			
with dexamethasone	8/8	1/4	9/12 (75%)
with placebo	3/5	2/3	5/8 (62.5%)
Response in points not on treatment			
with dexamethasone	2/5	2/4	4/9 (44%)
with placebo	2/4	1/2	3/6(50%)
Response on or off treatment			
with dexamethasone	10/13	3/8	13/21 (62%)
with placebo	5/9	3/5	8/14 (57%)

[a] Chemotherapy within 28 days of study.

to receive dexamethasone in the first treatment arm, and three of the five patients randomized to placebo).

Of the two patients who had not responded at Day 5, one patient subsequently responded to dexamethasone in the second treatment phase.

Ten patients were not 'on treatment' at time of study (no chemotherapy within 28 days). Nine were evaluable for response (one patient having died at Day 3). Four of these patients showed resolution of their obstruction by Day 5 (two out of five on dexamethasone, and two out of four on placebo).

Of the two patients on placebo who did not respond, one responded to dexamethasone during the second treatment period. Of the three patients on dexamethasone who did not respond, one subsequently responded to dexamethasone 'off study'.

Of the total 22 patients evaluable for response, 15 'responded' (five on placebo, 10 on dexamethasone). Twelve of the 15 responders remained out of complete obstruction at Day 10.

Trial 2

Fourteen patients were randomized in this study and all commenced the study. Nine patients were randomized to receive dexamethasone and five to receive placebo. Of the 14 patients, 13 are evaluable for response (one patient was withdrawn at Day 2 because of toxicity, see Table 10.2).

Seven patients were 'on treatment' (chemotherapy within 28 days of study). Three of these patients had resolution of their obstruction by Day 5 (one out of four randomized to dexamethasone and two out of the three patients randomized to placebo). All responses were maintained to Day 10. Of the four nonresponding patients, two subsequently responded after crossover (one on placebo, one on dexamethasone).

Six patients were classed as 'off treatment' (no chemotherapy within 28 days). Three of these had resolution of their obstruction at Day 5 (two out of four on dexamethasone, one out of two on placebo). None of the patients who remained in obstruction at Day 5 had resolved at Day 10, and one patient who had responded had reobstructed by Day 10. Of the total 13 evaluable patients, six responded (three out of eight on dexamethasone and three out of five on placebo).

When both studies are combined, 35 patients are evaluable for response. Twenty-one out of the 35 (60 per cent) showed resolution of their obstruction by Day 5. Eight of the total 14 patients randomized to placebo (57 per cent) and 13 of the 21 randomized to dexamethasone (62 per cent) responded.

Toxicity proved difficult to differentiate from symptoms of the underlying condition. Apart from the one patient who was withdrawn because of gastrointestinal toxicity, there were few side-effects that could definitely be attributable to the study drug. Several patients commented on an unpleasant perianal sensation when receiving intravenous dexamethasone.

Discussion

Research in patients with advanced malignant disease is difficult. The patients are often unwell and may already have been subjected to multiple trials during the course of their disease. Attrition rates are high and it is not unusual for patients to fail to complete studies because of a deterioration in their general condition. The staff often have a negative attitude to the thought of subjecting dying patients to any more experimentation. On the other hand, there is very little 'science' behind many of the treatments used in palliative care and many patients are subjected to symptomatic treatments with well-documented side-effects, but unproved benefit. Many of the 'standard' drugs used routinely in palliative care have been 'ushered in' because of common usage and not because of any proof of their effectiveness.[10]

The use of dexamethasone in bowel obstruction is a case in point. Corticosteroids are not without side-effects. Dyspepsia, hyperglycaemia, sleep disturbance, psychic change, proximal myopathy and weight gain are all well recognized and not uncommon side-effects,[11] as are more serious gastrointestinal side-effects (e.g. peptic ulceration, gut perforation), especially with higher doses.[12] Steroids do have many non-specific benefits, however, in the form of improved mood, general well-being and appetite stimulation.[13,14] Similarly, they are known to reduce tumour-associated inflammation[15] and this activity is used to great benefit in the palliation of symptoms such as those associated with raised intracranial pressure, airway obstruction, carcinomatosis lymphangitis and cord-compression.[16,17] It would seem logical, therefore, that dexamethasone might speed up resolution of a malignant bowel obstruction by reducing gut wall oedema. This has never been proven, however, and despite the side-effects, the use of dexamethasone has become almost standard practice, at least in this hospital, for the medical management of bowel obstruction.

These studies were designed in an attempt to answer the question as to the place of steroids in malignant bowel obstruction. The patients were stratified according to whether or not they were receiving chemotherapy. Bowel obstruction is not uncommon in patients on active treatment and to exclude these patients would have made it even more difficult to accrue sufficient numbers. Both studies were abandoned, however, having failed to reach accrual targets, despite being undertaken in a large cancer centre which sees many cases of malignant bowel obstruction each year.

The first study suggested a trend towards the beneficial effect of corticosteroids, but the chances of resolution of bowel obstruction appeared to be largely determined by whether or not the patient was on chemotherapy. This might be because these patients were more likely to be at an earlier stage of their disease and, therefore, have a smaller tumour 'load'. This may be a greater determinant of resolution of a bowel obstruction than any effect of dexamethasone. The aetiology of the obstruction may be different in this scenario, that is secondary to inflammation and oedema of the bowel wall rather than to obstruction by a large tumour mass.

The small sample size in the first study dictates that the power of any comparison between groups would be very low. In Trial 2, no evidence of any effect of either being 'on treatment' or of the use of dexamethasone is observed and the number of patients is even less. Unfortunately, due to the small number of patients in each of the trials and the added stratification by treatment, it has not been possible to make a meaningful overall formal statistical statement. Classical methods which allow combination of data across studies require larger numbers than available here, such that the two trials could not be formally analysed as one although the combined results have been shown in Table 10.2. We are currently unable to prove or disprove any effect that dexamethasone may have in the resolution of bowel obstruction. To prove that the difference in response rate shown in this study was significant (i.e. that there is a 5 per cent difference in response rate between dexamethasone (62 per cent) and placebo (57 per cent)), 4000 patients would have to be randomized. If we wished to prove a 20 per cent difference, assuming a response rate of 50 per cent to placebo and 70 per cent to dexamethasone, 260 patients would be required.

Practical difficulties in conducting this trial included the difficulty in differentiating partial from complete obstruction, a reluctance by some to submit palliative care patients to iv therapy and the possibility of receiving a placebo and the recruitment of patients presenting at night and at weekends.

Probably the major factor in the failure of recruitment to this trial, however, was the belief on the part of many of the attending physicians and nursing staff that dexamethasone has an established role in the management of bowel obstruction. This belief has never been substantiated but, as the use of steroids has become almost routine (at least in this centre), it is unlikely that the definitive trial can now ever be done. This is particularly unfortunate when one considers that this condition may resolve spontaneously (as illustrated by the patients receiving placebo in this study) and that the potential side-effects of corticosteroids are well known. It is notable, however, that neither of these studies identified any side-effect that was intolerable or which might not be attributable to the underlying disease.

This work also illustrates the dismal prognosis of patients with malignant bowel obstruction, the median survival from obstruction to death in both studies being about two months. This supports a previous study by Piver and colleagues[18] which reports a 2.5 month median survival in 60 women with intestinal obstruction from ovarian cancer referred for surgery. The median survival following surgery for bowel obstruction has been reviewed by Ripamonti[19] and ranges from 2.0 to 11.0 months.

Despite the lack of supporting benefit, our recommendation would still be that it is reasonable to subject a patient with malignant bowel obstruction to a 'trial' of dexamethasone; it may speed resolution, provide non-specific benefit (improved general well-being) and is unlikely to do any harm. The therapeutic trial should not be continued for more than five days, however, if no benefit is seen. With the development of new agents such as octreotide for use in bowel obstruction,[20,21] it is unlikely that a definitive trial of dexamethasone versus placebo in malignant bowel obstruction will now ever be carried out.

References

1 Baines, M., Oliver, D.J. and Carter, R.L. (1985) Medical management of intestinal obstruction in patients with advanced malignant disease. *Lancet*, 2: 990–3.
2 Chan, A. and Woodruff, R.K. (1992) Intestinal obstruction in patients with widespread intra-abdominal malignancy. *Journal of Pain Symptom Management*, 7: 339–42.
3 Fainsinger, R.L., Spachynzki, K., Hanson, J. and Bruera, E. (1994) Symptom control in terminally ill patients with malignant bowel obstruction. *Journal of Pain Symptom Management*, 9: 12–18.
4 Ripamonti, C. (1994) Management of bowel obstruction in advanced cancer patients. *Journal of Pain Symptom Management*, 9: 193–200.
5 Fainsinger, R.L. *et al.* (1994) Op. cit.
6 Ripamonti, C. (1994) Op. cit.

7 Reid, D.B. (1988) Palliative management of bowel obstruction. *The Medical Journal of Australia*, 148: 54.
8 Baines, M. (1993) The pathophysiology and management of malignant intestinal obstruction, in D. Doyle, G. Hanks and N. MacDonald (eds) *Oxford Textbook of Palliative Medicine*. Oxford: Oxford Medical Publications, 311–16.
9 Twycross, R. (1992) Corticosteroids in advanced cancer. *British Medical Journal*, 305: 969–70.
10 Eddy, D.M. (1993) Three battles to watch in the 1990s. *Journal of the American Medical Association*, 270: 520–6.
11 Twycross, R. (1992) Op. cit.
12 Heidmal, K., Hirschberg, H., Slettebo, H., Watne, K. and Nome, O. (1992) High incidence of serious side effects of high-dose dexamethasone treatment in patients with epidural spinal cord compression. *Journal of Neurooncology*, 12: 141–4.
13 Bruera, E., Roca, E., Cedaro, L., Carraro, S. and Chacon, R. (1985) Action of oral methyl prednisolone in terminal cancer patients: a prospective randomised double-blind study. *Cancer Treatment Reports*, 69: 751–4.
14 Popiela, T., Lucchi, R. and Giongo, F. (1989) Methylprednisolone as palliative therapy for female terminal cancer patients. *British Journal of Cancer and Clinical Oncology*, 25: 1823–9.
15 Bodsch, W., Rommel, T., Ophoff, B.G. and Menzel, J. (1987) Factors responsible for retention of fluid in human tumour oedema and the effect of dexamethasone. *Journal of Neurosurgery*, 67: 250–7.
16 Koehler, P.J. (1995) Use of corticosteroids in neuro-oncology. *Anticancer Drugs*, 6: 19–33.
17 Ahmedzai, S. (1993) Palliation of respiratory symptoms, in D. Doyle, G. Hanks and N. MacDonald (eds) *Oxford Textbook of Palliative Medicine*. Oxford: Oxford Medical Publications.
18 Piver, M.S., Barlow, J.J., Shashikant, B., Lele, M.D. and Frank, A. (1982) Survival after ovarian cancer induced intestinal obstruction. *Gynecological Oncology*, 13: 44–9.
19 Ripamonti, C. (1994) Op. cit.
20 Mercadante, S., Spoldi, E., Caraceni, A., Maddaloni, S. and Simonetti, M.T. (1993) Octreotide in relieving gastrointestinal symptoms due to bowel obstruction. *Palliative Medicine*, 7: 295–9.
21 Khoo, D., Hall, E., Motson, R., Riley, J., Denman, K. and Waxman, J. (1994) Palliation of malignant intestinal obstruction using octreotide. *European Journal of Cancer Care*, 30: 28–30.

Acknowledgement

Hardy, J., Ling, J., Mansi, J. *et al.* (1998) Pitfalls in placebo-controlled trials in palliative care: dexamethasone for the palliation of malignant bowel obstruction. *Palliative Medicine*, 12: 437–42.

11

Multicentre randomized controlled trial of nursing intervention for breathlessness in patients with lung cancer

MARY BREDIN, JESSICA CORNER,
MEINIR KRISHNASAMY, HILARY PLANT,
CHRIS BAILEY, ROGER A'HERN

Introduction

Breathlessness is increasingly recognized as not simply a symptom of disordered breathing but also a complex interplay of physical, psychological, emotional, and functional factors.[1] Between 10 per cent and 15 per cent of patients with lung cancer have breathlessness at diagnosis, and 65 per cent will have the symptom at some point during their illness.[2] Alongside cough, it is the symptom most frequently reported by patients with lung cancer.[3] The subjective experience of breathlessness may not be directly related to the extent of the disease. Factors such as anxiety can play an important part in exacerbating the symptom, and this is particularly evident in the context of an imminently life-threatening illness such as lung cancer.[4]

Pharmacological and non-pharmacological interventions for breathlessness have not been evaluated. Although recognized palliative interventions are used, breathlessness remains unrelieved.[5]

Corner and colleagues set out to identify and evaluate nursing strategies for managing breathlessness and adopted an integrated approach that emphasized the importance of not separating psychological and physical aspects of the symptom.[6] They developed a therapeutic intervention that aimed to increase fitness and tolerance of restricted lung function and reduce functional disability while acknowledging the meaning of breathlessness in the context of life threatening illness. In a small randomized controlled study, distress caused by breathlessness was reduced and functional ability and ability to perform activities of daily living increased.[7] A larger multicentre study was organized to evaluate the effect of the intervention on a larger, more diverse sample and to establish the feasibility of integrating the new approach in a range of treatment centres.

Methods

Study design

This multicentre study was coordinated from the Macmillan Practice Development Unit at the Centre for Cancer and Palliative Care Studies, Institute of Cancer Research, London. Patients diagnosed with small cell lung cancer, non-small cell lung cancer or mesothelioma who had completed treatment and reported breathlessness were invited to take part in the study. Entry criteria for the study defined shortness of breath as a reported change in breathing or a degree of breathlessness as perceived by the patient and reported as a problem that caused distress.

In each of the participating centres, once a patient from one of the participating centres had consented to take part in the trial, a telephone call was made to the Institute of Cancer Research's clinical trials office, which was responsible for independent randomization to either intervention or control groups. The trials office informed the participating centre which group the patient had been assigned to. The patient was then asked to confirm whether he or she remained happy to participate in the study. Patients in the control group were given standard care and also had their breathlessness and its effects on life monitored; patients in the intervention group attended a nursing clinic. In the nursing clinics, patients received a package of interventions tailored to individual patients (see box) aimed at helping them to cope with breathlessness and maximize their existing lung

---

Box 11.1   Intervention carried out by specialist nurses

- Detailed assessment of breathlessness and factors that ameliorate or exacerbate it
- Advice and support for patients and their families on ways of managing breathlessness
- Exploration of the meaning of breathlessness, their disease, and feelings about the future
- Training in breathing control techniques, progressive muscle relaxation, and distraction exercises
- Goal setting to complement breathing and relaxation techniques, to help in the management of functional and social activities, and to support the development and adoption of coping strategies
- Early recognition of problems warranting pharmacological or medical intervention

function. Many of these strategies are commonly used in settings for patients with chronic lung diseases but are not routinely used with lung cancer patients. Best supportive care was defined as the standard management and treatment for breathlessness available to patients within each centre. This included pharmacological and palliative treatments and treatment of associated problems such as anxiety and depression. All patients taking part had access to all routinely available supportive care.

Patients in the intervention group were invited to attend the nursing clinic once a week for up to eight weeks (and for not less than three weeks). Data were collected from both groups at Weeks 1, 4, and 8. An independent data monitoring committee was set up to advise on the conduct of the study.

Recruitment of centres

Six hospital centres from around the United Kingdom volunteered to join the study. Each centre was granted ethical approval from its local research ethics committee. Informed written consent was obtained from patients, who were also aware of their ability to withdraw from the study at any time. All nurses taking part were taught the intervention in the same way, using a practice guideline, and the correct delivery of the intervention was monitored.

Outcome measures

Several self-completed outcome measures were used to assess the effects of the intervention. Patients' subjective experience of breathlessness was assessed with visual analogue scales measuring breathlessness at worst and at best and distress due to breathlessness. The primary outcome measure was distress due to breathlessness. Other measures included the WHO performance status scale,[8] the hospital anxiety and depression scale,[9] and the Rotterdam symptom checklist.[10]

Statistical methods

Data from the research interviews and assessment instruments were entered onto EXCEL and SPSS–PC. As the data were not normally distributed, descriptive statistics and the non-parametric Mann-Whitney test were used in the analysis. The intended accrual was 150 patients to detect a difference in the proportion of patients who showed an improvement over eight weeks, corresponding to 10 per cent showing an improvement in one group and 30 per cent in the other, or 25 per cent in one group and 50 per cent in the other (approximate 90 per cent power, 5 per cent two-sided significance level). (See Chapter 3 for an explanation of power and significance levels). In the final sample of 100 patients the power would be 70–75 per cent.

At the outset of the study the principal time point chosen for analysis was from baseline to eight weeks; we assumed that this was when the intervention would show its maximum impact.[11] Patients who withdrew from the study for any reason other than that they reported being too well to continue were given a change score that was one more (that is, worse) than the maximum of the patients who did not withdraw. Similarly, any patient who withdrew because he or she reported being too well to continue was given a score which was one less than the minimum score of the patients who did not withdraw. This method of treating withdrawals is recommended by Gould,[12] who ranked patients who withdraw for reasons other than an improvement in their condition below patients who did not withdraw, and ranked those who withdrew because they improved above those who did not withdraw.

Results

A total of 119 patients were recruited to the study. One centre failed to adhere to the trial protocol, and data for its 16 patients were excluded on the advice of the data monitoring committee (an audit of data indicated that control patients from the centre also received strategies identified as being part of the intervention). At baseline the intervention group (51 patients) and the control group (52 patients) were similar in terms of age, sex, diagnosis and metastatic disease and the outcome measurements for the groups did not differ significantly (Table 11.1).

Sixteen patients died during the course of the study and 28 patients withdrew. Of the 27 patients who withdrew but did not report an improvement in their breathlessness, 16 withdrew because of a deterioration in their condition (13 control, three intervention, exact P = 0.01) and four were unhappy with the arm to which they had been allocated (three control, one intervention). This left seven patients who withdrew for other reasons (two control, five intervention). The major difference in the number of withdrawals between the groups therefore occurred where the patient's condition deteriorated. This was also reflected by the fact that the survival of the patients who withdrew from the control arm was significantly worse than the survival of patients withdrawing from the intervention arm (hazard ratio 2.5, P < 0.05, excluding the intervention patient who withdrew because he felt better). Survival of all withdrawals versus non-withdrawals was also significantly worse (hazard ratio 2.0, P < 0.01). All withdrawing patients or those who died were assumed to have a poor outcome relative to all the patients for whom an eight-week assessment was available.

Table 11.1   Baseline data for intervention and control groups

Questionnaire	Intervention group		Control group	
	No. of patients	Median (range)	No. of patients	Median (range)
Visual analogue scale:				
Distress caused by breathlessness	47	6 (0–10)	49	5 (0–10)
Breathlessness at worst	47	7.5 (0–10)	49	7.9 (0–10)
Breathlessness at best	47	4 (0–9.1)	49	3.5 (0–8.9)
WHO performance status	49	2 (0–3)	51	1 (0–3)
Hospital anxiety and depression scale:				
Anxiety	48	7 (0–17)	49	6 (0–17)
Depression	48	6 (0–16)	49	5 (2–14)
Rotterdam symptom checklist:				
Psychological symptoms	48	14 (7–27)	49	14 (7–26)
Physical symptoms	48	50 (34–77)	49	49 (30–77)
Activity (total items 38–44)	45	12 (7–26)	49	12 (7–27)
Activity (subitems R41, R43, R44)	45	6 (3–12)	49	5 (3–12)
Quality of life	45	3 (1–6)	49	3 (1–6)

Scores of patients who died were not included in this analysis. In several cases data were missing because patients did not complete individual questions on the questionnaires.

As overall survival of the two groups of patients did not differ significantly, it cannot be concluded that the intervention improved survival. However, the pattern of mortality showed that the intervention patients may have had improved survival over the first six months, but this was not maintained. No appreciable differences in medication between the two groups were found. The proportion of patients taking opioids in intervention group patients at baseline was 22 per cent and at eight weeks 27 per cent, the corresponding figures for the control group were 23 per cent and 33 per cent (the respective percentages for other medications were: steroids–intervention 31 per cent and 45 per cent, control 27 per cent and 30 per cent; bronchodilators – intervention 27 per cent and 27 per cent, control 31 per cent and 44 per cent; non-opioid analgesics – intervention 51 per cent and 33 per cent, control 44 per cent and 55 per cent; antibiotics – intervention 5 per cent and 15 per cent, control 2 per cent and 11 per cent; and psychotropics – intervention 14 per cent and 18 per cent, control 17 per cent and 22 per cent).

At baseline both groups reported high levels of distress due to breathlessness and associated functional impairment (Table 11.2). At eight weeks, the intervention group showed significant improvement for breathlessness at best, WHO performance status, levels of depression, and physical symptom distress. Levels of anxiety and distress due to breathlessness improved slightly. Activity levels did not differ (P = 0.10). The groups were similar

Table 11.2 Change between baseline and eight weeks in intervention and control groups in scores

| Questionnaire | Intervention group | | Control group | | |
	No. of patients	Median (range) change	No. of patients	Median (range) change	P value
Visual analogue scales:					
Distress caused by breathlessness	49	0 (–9–11)	51	10 (–7–11)	0.09
Breathlessness at worst	50	1 (–7.2–8.5)	52	4.8 (–6.2–8.5)	0.14
Breathlessness at best	50	1.3 (–7.1–8)	52	7.0 (–3.3–8)	0.03
WHO performance status	51	0 (–3–3)	52	2 (–1–3)	0.02
Hospital anxiety and depression:					
Anxiety	50	0 (–7–11)	52	9.5 (–6–11)	0.08
Depression	50	0.5 (–10–7)	52	6 (–7–7)	0.02
Rotterdam symptom checklist:					
Psychological symptoms	50	1 (–9–13)	52	9 (–8–13)	0.21
Physical symptoms	50	2.5 (–24–16)	52	14 (–11–16)	0.04
Activity:					
Items 38–44	47	2 (–12–15)	52	8.5 (–4–15)	0.1
Subitems R41, R43, R44	47	0 (–6–9)	52	5.5 (–3–9)	0.05
Quality of life (1 item)	47	1 (–4–4)	52	2 (–2–4)	0.25

Negative scores show improvement.

in breathlessness at worst, psychological distress, and overall global quality of life.

Discussion

Breathlessness in advanced lung cancer is an unpleasant and intractable problem that directly interferes with all aspects of daily living and can provoke intense anxiety.[13] Patients may also receive little or no help or advice on how to cope during attacks of breathlessness.[14] This is the first multicentre randomized controlled study that set out to evaluate nursing strategies for managing breathlessness in various treatment centres in the United Kingdom. The findings show that patients attending nursing clinics for breathlessness experienced improvements in breathlessness, performance status, and physical and emotional states.

Precisely how the intervention affects depression and anxiety is unclear. Changes from baseline to eight weeks in scores on the hospital anxiety and depression scale suggest a general improvement in mood for the intervention group. Two particular elements of the intervention might be responsible for the improvements: the emphasis on teaching more effective ways of coping with breathlessness and the opportunity to talk about difficult feelings and concerns.

Possible criticisms

The analysis rested on the assumption that patients who withdrew from the study had a poor outcome; clearly, it would have been preferable if their outcomes had actually been assessed. The method of analysis also assumed that all patients were able to show a change in either direction on the rating scales, but patients whose baseline measurements were at the extremes of a scale would be able to show change in only one direction. As the groups were similar at baseline, however, both groups should have been affected equally by this problem. Though the analysis of such a large number of outcomes would imply that one or two might be significant by chance even if the intervention had no effect, five out of 11 outcomes reached conventional levels of significance and all outcomes favoured the intervention group. Though the differences between the two groups were significant, the magnitude of the effect of intervention is more difficult to assess, and data need to be interpreted with caution. Not all patients benefited, but performance status gives an idea of the degree of benefit some patients experienced. The median change for the intervention group was 0: this group maintained the ability to carry out activities. For the control group there was a median deterioration of two points, so that for patients at baseline whose score was 2 (that is, up and about for 50 per cent of waking hours, and capable of self-care) typically deteriorated to grade 4 at eight weeks (that is, confined to bed or chair, no self-care, completely disabled).

Conclusion

This study set out to evaluate a nursing intervention for breathlessness in patients with lung cancer and to replicate a previous study.[15] Most patients who managed to complete the study had a poor prognosis, and breathlessness was typically a symptom of their deteriorating condition. Considering the difficulties of randomizing very ill patients to an eight-week intervention study, the completion and results of this study are an achievement in the field of palliative care. The results confirm the findings from the earlier study and show that intervention based on psychosocial support, breathing control, and coping strategies can help patients deal with their breathlessness.

References

1 O'Driscoll, M. and Corner, J. (1999) The experience of breathlessness in lung cancer. *European Journal of Cancer Care*, 8: 37–43.
2 Twycross, R.G. and Lack, S.A. (1986) *Therapeutics in Terminal Cancer*. Edinburgh: Churchill Livingstone.

3 Muers, M.F. and Round, C.E. (1993) Palliation of symptoms in non-small cell lung cancer: a study by the Yorkshire Regional Cancer Organisation Thoracic Group. *Thorax*, 48: 339–43.
4 Corner, J., Plant, H. and Warner, L. (1995) Developing a nursing approach to managing dyspnoea in lung cancer. *International Journal of Palliative Nursing*, 1: 5–10.
5 Higginson, I. and McCarthy, M. (1989) Measuring symptoms in terminal cancer: are pain and dyspnoea controlled? *Journal of the Royal Society of Medicine of London*, 82: 264–7.
6 Corner, J. *et al.* (1995) Op. cit.
7 Corner, J., Plant, H., A'Hern, R. and Bailey, C. (1996) Non-pharmacological intervention for breathlessness in lung cancer. *Palliative Medicine*, 10: 299–305.
8 World Health Organization (1979) *WHO Handbook for Reporting Results of Cancer Treatment* (WHO offset publication No. 48). Geneva: WHO.
9 Zigmond, A.S. and Snaith, R.P. (1979) The hospital anxiety and depression scale. *Acta Psychiatrica Scandinavica*, 67: 361–70.
10 De Haes, J., Olschewski, M., Fayers, P. *et al.* (1996) *The Rotterdam symptom checklist (RSCL): a manual.* Groningen: Northern Centre for Healthcare Research, University of Groningen.
11 Corner, J. *et al.* (1996) Op. cit.
12 Gould, A.L. (1980) A new approach to the analysis of clinical drug trials with withdrawals. *Biometrics*, 36: 721–7.
13 Corner, J. *et al.* (1996) Op. cit.
14 Roberts, D., Thorne, S.E. and Person, C. (1993) The experience of dyspnoea in late stage cancer: patients and nurses' perspectives. *Cancer Nursing*, 16: 310–20.
15 Corner, J. *et al.* (1996) Op. cit.

Acknowledgements

We thank Macmillan Cancer Relief for funding this study, Professor Mike Richards and Dr Tim Sheard for advice on the conduct of the study, and the staff of the Clinical Trials Statistics Unit, Institute of Cancer Research, Sutton, Surrey, for providing an independent randomization service. We especially thank and acknowledge the Macmillan and specialist nurses at the six participating centres: Sian Dennison, Tony Shute, and Glad Baldry, Plymouth Hospitals NHS Trust; Jo O'Neill, Neil Cliffe Cancer Care Charity, and Michael Connolly, Wythenshawe Hospital, Manchester; Diane Stidston, Anna Farrar, and Jane McKay, Norfolk and Norwich Healthcare NHS Trust; Rachel Hornsby, Kathy Penn, and Anne Noble, Southampton University Hospitals Trust, Cancer Care Directorate; Brian Lowden and Norma Thomson, Hove General Hospital, Brighton Healthcare NHS Trust; Kay Doyle and Simon Jones, Tenovus Cancer Information Centre/Llandough Hospital, Cardiff.

This article was first published in the *British Medical Journal*, Bredin, M., Corner, J., Plant, H., Bailey, C. and O'Hearn, A. (1999) Multicentre study of nursing intervention for breathlessness in lung cancer, 3: 901–4, and is reproduced by permission of the *British Medical Journal*.

12

Outcome measures in palliative care for advanced cancer patients: a review

JULIE HEARN AND IRENE J. HIGGINSON

Introduction

In the context of health and illness, outcome is usually defined in terms of the achievement or failure to achieve desired goals.[1] The measurement of the health outcome of interventions can be linked to the assessment of the appropriateness of health care interventions.[2] The use of outcome measures can therefore help determine whether a method of treatment or particular intervention package is worthwhile.[3] Consequently, measurement of this 'attributable effect of intervention or its lack on a previous state of health'[4] has important implications for the purchasing of health care services.

Outcome measures in palliative care for patients with advanced cancer require the measurement of aspects that reflect the specific goals of palliative care, such as improving the quality of life before death, controlling symptoms and supporting the family.[5] Measuring the effectiveness of palliative care interventions is becoming increasingly important[6] because it allows the evaluation and development of effective and efficacious palliative care teams.

A variety of clinical audit tools and systems for palliative care have been developed in recent years, but these are being used in various ways and are constantly changing or being supplemented by new measures. This review aimed to identify and examine outcome measures that have been used, or proposed for use in the clinical audit of palliative care of patients with advanced cancer, and to assess these systematically using well-defined criteria.

Method

Sources of literature

Database searches were performed using MEDLINE (1991–5), CANCERLIT (1991–5), Healthplan (1985–95), and 'Oncolink' on the Internet (The University of Pennsylvania Cancer Center Resource, 1994–6). The search terms used, either singly or in combination, were audit, palliative care, hospice care, terminal care, clinical or medical or nursing audit, quality assurance, audit measures, assessment and outcome. Further measures were located with the assistance of a multiprofessional steering group, through personal communications with other professionals working in palliative care, and from an investigation of the grey literature. New measures published during the review period were also identified.

Inclusion criteria

The criteria for inclusion were:

1 that the target population included cancer patients, or patients with advanced disease receiving palliative care, or considered by the authors to be appropriate for this patient group;
2 the measure contained more than one domain; and
3 the measure could be used on patients with all cancer types.

Measures that have been used in cancer care but were specific to a particular patient group, for example, leukaemia patients (Cancer Leukaemia Group B Studies – CALGB), or measures which concentrated on only one life domain, for example, physical symptoms (McGill Pain Questionnaire), were excluded from the review (see Bowling).[7] It was also important to identify only those measures that had been used for patients receiving palliative care or proposed for use measuring outcomes at this stage of the disease trajectory. For example, measures specifically designed to assess the outcome of non-palliative cancer chemotherapy, such as the Breast Cancer Chemotherapy Questionnaire (BCCQ), were not included.[8]

Assessment of identified measures

Measures were then assessed following the criteria outlined in Table 12.1.[9] Content validity was further assessed by whether the measure covered the particular domains reported to be relevant to palliative care (physical, psychological and spiritual dimensions), and how many items were contained in each domain.

Table 12.1   Criteria used to assess outcome measures

Validity – the instrument measures what it intends to measure
Content validity – does the measure cover those domains considered important?
Criterion validity – does the measure correlate with superior measures or predict future outcome?
Construct validity – does the measure conform with the results using other established scales (or discriminate between groups of patients)?

Reliability – the instrument produces the same results when repeated on an unchanged population
Inter-rater reliability – does the measure produce similar results when used by different observers?
Test–retest reliability – does the measure produce similar results when used at different points in time?
Internal consistency – do individual items within the instrument correlate with each other?

Responsiveness to change – the instrument is able to detect clinically significant change
Has the measure demonstrated change as part of a clinical trial or cohort follow-up?
Does the measure discriminate between differing degrees of disease severity?

Appropriateness of format – the instrument is suitable for its intended use

---

Source: Ramsey, M., Winget, C. and Higginson, I. (1995) Review: measures to determine the outcome of community services for people with dementia. *Age and Ageing*, 24 (1): 75–83.

Results

In total, 41 measures were identified (see Tables 12.2 and 12.3). Twelve of these satisfied the inclusion criteria. These measures contained between five and 56 items and covered the physical, psychological and spiritual domains of life to differing extents (see Table 12.3).

To summarize the 12 measures: three are completed by a professional;[10–12] seven by the patient himself or herself;[13–19] two contain both patient and professional completion elements;[20,21] eight assess items relating only to the patient,[22–29] whereas four may also consider the family or carer unit;[30–33] seven have been validated in just one setting;[34–40] five contain 30 or more items;[41–45] two were designed for the assessment of clinical trial interventions.[46,47] This chapter will now describe each of these measures in more detail.

Table 12.2   Scales used in the assessment of the quality of life of cancer patients

---

The World Health Organization (WHO) Functional Scale
The Zubrod Scale
The Eastern Co-operative Oncology Group Performance Scale (ECOGP)
The McGill Pain Questionnaire (MPG)
Lasry Sexual Functioning Scale for Breast Cancer Patients
WHO Symptom Checklist
Medical Research Council (MRC) UK Scale
The Qualitator
Functional Assessment of Cancer Therapy (FACT-G)
Functional Living Index – Cancer (FLIC)
Cancer Inventory of Problem Situations (CIPS)
Cancer Rehabilitation Evaluation System (CARES)
Spitzer Quality of Life (QL) Index
Linear Analogue Self-Assessment (LASA) Scale
Ontario Cancer Institute–Royal Marsden Linear Analogue Self-Assessment Scale
Padilla Quality of Life (QL) Scale
Multidimensional Quality of Life Scale (MQOLS-CA)
Holmes and Dickerson
Global Quality of Life Scales (Coates)
Quality of Life Index
Breast Cancer Chemotherapy Questionnaire (BCCQ)
Visual Analogue Scale (VAS) for Bone Marrow Transplant Patients
European Neuroblastoma Study Group Quality of Life Assessment Form – Children
   (QLAF-C)
Cancer Leukaemia Group B Studies (CALGB)
Ability Index
Burge Quality of Life Severity Scale
Anamnestic Comparative Self-Assessment (ACSA)
WHO Quality of Life Assessment Instrument (WHOQOL)
TWiST

Source: Bowling, A. (1994) *Measuring Disease: A Review of Disease-specific Quality of Life Measurement Scales*. Buckingham: Open University Press.

An initial assessment of suffering[48]

This measure was developed on 259 advanced cancer patients in acute hospitals. A five-point Likert Scale with scores ranging from five for 'good' to one for 'bad' was used to record the answers to the 43 questions either by the patient unaided or by a trained nurse interviewer. The questions have been refined to give a shorter 20-item questionnaire suitable for use during the initial assessment by a member of any profession in the hospice or palliative care team.

Table 12.3 Measures for assessing the outcome of palliative care for people with advanced cancer

Name of measure (author and year)	Number of items and domains covered	Validity	Reliability	Responsiveness to change	Appropriateness of format			
					Setting	Time	Administration	
An Initial Assessment of Suffering[a]	43 (patient); mood, symptoms, fears and family worries, knowledge and involvement, support	correlates with Spitzer Quality of Life Index physical health groups	internal consistency	stable over time	in-patient	not known	patient completion or by professional interview	
Edmonton Symptom Assessment Schedule – ESAS[b]	9 (patient); pain activity, nausea, depression, anxiety, drowsiness, appetite, well-being, shortness of breath	correlates with STAS (except for activity)	inter-rater (0.5–0.9)	improvement demonstrated in palliative care	in-patient	few minutes	patient completion or with nurse assistance	
European Organisation for Research on Treatment of Cancer – EORTC QLQ-C30[c]	30 (patient); 9 multi-item scales including 5 functional, 3 symptom scales and a global quality of life scale	inter-scale correlation, correlates with clinical status	internal consistency (0.54–0.86)	palliative care module being evaluated in Europe	outpatient	11–12 minutes	patient completion	
Hebrew Rehabilitation Centre for Aged Quality of Life Index – HRCA-QL[d]	5 (patient); mobility, daily living, health, attitude, support	correlates with Uni and Multi scale version and with the Karnofsky Performance Index	internal consistency (0.77) and inter-rater (0.6–0.81)	scores correlate with survival	community in-patient	1–2 minutes	professional completion	

Table 12.3 *(cont'd)*

Name of measure (author and year)	Number of items and domains covered	Validity	Reliability	Responsiveness to change	Appropriateness of format			Administration
					Setting	Time		
The McGill Quality of Life Questionnaire – MQOL[e]	17 (patient); physical symptoms, psychological symptoms, outlook on life and meaningful existence	correlates with Spitzer Quality of Life and SIS	internal consistency (0.89)	distinguishes between patients	in-patient outpatient	not known		patient completion
The McMaster Quality of Life Scale – MQLS[f]	32 (patient); physical symptoms, functional status, social functioning, emotional status, cognition, sleep and rest, energy and vitality, general life satisfaction, meaning of life	correlates with Spitzer Quality of Life	internal consistency (0.62–0.79) inter-rater (0.83–0.95)	changes in scores were related to whether the patient felt they had changed	community in-patient outpatient	patients 3–30 minutes, staff under 3 minutes, family approximately 3 minutes		patient, family or staff completion
Palliative Care Assessment – PACA	12 (patient and relatives); symptom control, insight and future placement	the symptom scores correlate with the McCorkle symptom distress scale	inter-rater (0.44–1)	improvement demonstrated in palliative care	in-patient	few minutes		professional completion
Palliative Care Core Standards – PCCS[g]	6 core standards and 56 process and outcome items (patient and carer); symptom control, information, support, bereavement care and emotional support, specialist education for staff	currently being tested	currently being tested	not evaluated as yet	in-patient	expected to take about 10 minutes		professional, patient, carer and the bereaved

Instrument	Number of items and content	Validity	Reliability	Sensitivity	Setting	Time	Completion
Rotterdam Symptom Checklist – RSCL[h]	34 (patient); physical and psychosocial symptoms	inter-scale correlation for psychological dimension, less for physical distress items	internal consistency (0.82–0.88)	not evaluated	outpatient	8 minutes	complete separate questionnaires-patient completion
Support Team Assessment Schedule – STAS[i]	17 (patient and carer); pain and symptom control, insight, psychosocial, family needs, planning affairs, home services communication, and support of other professionals	correlates with patient's and family's ratings and with HRCA-QL	inter-rater (0.65–0.94) internal consistency (0.68–0.89) test-retest (0.36–0.76)	improvement demonstrated in palliative care	community hospice	2 minutes	professional completion
Symptom Distress Scale – SDS[j]	13 (patient); nausea, mood, loss of appetite, insomnia, pain, mobility, fatigue, appearance, bowel pattern, concentration	correlates with global Quality of Life measures	internal consistency (0.78–0.89)	sensitive to changes in treatment over time	in-patient	not known	patient completion, in presence of an interviewer
The Schedule for the Evaluation of Individual Quality of Life – SEIQoL[k]	5 domains nominated by the individual; 30 hypothetical scenarios are rated based on these domains and weights are derived for each domain	correlates with McMaster health index questionnaire subscales for health status and physical function	internal consistency (0.48–0.74) internal validity (0.62–0.79)	does not distinguish between patients and controls pre-treatment	community in-patient	not known	patient completion as part of a structured interview

Notes:

a MacAdam, D.B. and Smith, M. (1987), see note 13.
b Bruera, E. *et al.* (1991), see note 14.
c Aaronson, N.K. *et al.* (1993), see note 15.
d Morris, J., Suissa, S., Sherwood, S. and Greer, D. (1986), see note 11.
e Cohen, S.R. *et al.* (1995), see note 16.
f Sterkenburg, C.A. and Woodward, C.A. (1996), see note 20.
g Trent Hospice Audit Group (1992), see note 21.
h de Haes, J.C.J.M. *et al.* (1990), see note 17.
i Morris, J. *et al.* (1986), see note 11.
j McCorkle, R. and Young, K. (1978), see note 18.
k O'Boyle, C.A. *et al.* (1994), see note 19.

Edmonton Symptom Assessment Schedule (ESAS)[49]

The ESAS was developed for quick assessment of outcomes in routine practice. This tool consists of nine Visual Analogue Scales (VASs). Patients draw a mark along a 100 mm line corresponding to how they feel, with the far left end of the line corresponding to the least degree of symptoms, and the far right 'worst' symptoms. The ESAS is completed on admission to hospital and twice daily thereafter by the patient, or with the assistance of a nurse. Patients who are unable to respond owing to cognitive failure are assessed by their nurse or a specially trained family member. The score for each item is recorded on a bar graph, allowing staff to visualize patterns of symptom control over time. Further testing of this measure's validity and reliability are required, particularly with reference to the potential bias introduced by a change in the person recording the answers on the VAS as care continues.

European Organisation for Research on Cancer Treatment (EORCT QLQ-C30)[50]

Developed with lung cancer patients to evaluate the quality of life of those patients participating in international clinical trials, this self-reporting questionnaire is both a reliable and valid measure of the quality of life of cancer patients in research settings. Questions cover the past week and responses are mainly in the format of a straightforward four-point Likert Scale, ranging from 1 for 'not at all' to 4 for 'very much'. It contains a generic core with cancer-specific modules and work is being carried out to extend the questionnaire for patients with more advanced cancer. At present, some questions are thought to be inappropriate for this patient group and have caused distress in patients with advanced disease in a French community setting (D. LaGabrielle, personal communication, 1995).

Hebrew Rehabilitation Centre for Aged Quality of Life (HRCA-QL)[51]

Adapted from the Spitzer Quality of Life Index (a scale developed for doctors to measure the quality of life of their cancer patients), with the item activity being replaced by mobility for the older target patient group. It has not been revalidated and has been criticized for lack of responsiveness in patients with advanced disease. Ratings for each item are scored from 0 to 2 to give a total score of 0–10 (higher scores equate to a better quality of life). It has been used to evaluate treatments and support services.

McGill Quality of Life Questionnaire (MQLO)[52]

Developed on advanced cancer patients treated at home or in an in-patient unit, the MQOL was designed to measure overall quality of life in people with a life-threatening illness and to indicate the areas in which the patient is doing well or poorly. The patient circles a number on a ten-point categorical scale, with the extremes of least desirable and most desirable at either end. It includes an existential domain which the authors propose plays a greater role in determining quality of life in patients with local or metastatic disease than in patients with no evidence of disease.

The McMaster Quality of Life Scale (MQLS)[53]

This measure was developed on 83 patients to measure the quality of life in a palliative patient population including cancer patients. Items are rated on a seven-point numerical scale with the direction of positive and negative descriptors varied. It is currently being refined and patients are now asked which ten items of the scale are most important to their quality of life. Patients who begin to experience difficulty filling in answers are then asked to rate only these ten, most important items.

Palliative Care Assessment (PACA)[54]

This measure was developed on 125 patients to assess the outcome of interventions made within two weeks of referral to a hospital palliative care team. The PACA form comprises three rating scales. Symptoms are scored on a four-point scale from 0 for 'absent' to 3 for 'daily life dominated by the symptom', assessing the severity of each symptom from the patient's perspective, using a semi-structured interview. Insight is assessed by an observer on a five-point scale, and plans for future care were asked of the patient and recorded on a four-point scale. Facilitation of the appropriate placement for hospital patients is a fundamental element of this measure.

Palliative Care Core Standards (PCCS)[55]

Originally a set of standards for in-patient hospice care and community teams, this tool has been refined and is currently being piloted in in-patient units as separate questionnaires for all those involved with the patient's well-being including the professionals, the patient and the carer. Structure, process, education and training are also covered, resulting in a comprehensive but lengthy tool at present.

Rotterdam Symptom Checklist (RSCL)[56]

Developed primarily as a tool to measure the symptoms reported by cancer patients participating in clinical research, this questionnaire uses a four-point Likert Scale to record responses on the bothersomeness of items over the last three days or week. Categories range from 'not at all' through to 'very much'. The authors suggest it may be useful in the evaluation of supportive care, but it may be inappropriate for patients to complete as disease advances.[57]

The Support Team Assessment Schedule (STAS)[58]

Developed for use with multidisciplinary cancer support teams, STAS is a validated measure of the effectiveness of palliative care.[59] Items were developed by cancer support teams to reflect the goals of palliative care. The effect of the items on the daily life of the patient over the last week is scored by a professional on a five-point Likert Scale ranging from 0 for 'none' (no effect) up to 4 for 'overwhelming effect'. STAS is widely used in community settings and has been adapted for use in in-patient settings and to assess individual symptoms.

The Symptom Distress Scale (SDS)[60]

This scale was developed for patients with a life-threatening disease, either cancer or heart disease, and can be used for all types of cancer. The scale is self-administered (usually in the presence of an interviewer), with responses rated on a five-point Likert Scale ranging from 1 for 'no distress' to 5 for 'extreme distress'. It concentrates mainly on the symptoms and mood in relation to quality of life.

Schedule for the Evaluation of Individual Quality of Life (SEIQoL)[61]

This measure was developed from the technique of 'judgement analysis' to measure patients' level of functioning. The measure allows respondents to nominate the five areas of life which are most important to them, rate their level of functioning or satisfaction with each, and indicate the relative importance of each area to their total quality of life. It has been tested in a variety of patient populations and healthy individuals, and has recently been reported for use clinically for patients with HIV or AIDS managed in general practice.

Discussion

In palliative care there are particular concerns about the use and relevance of outcome measures. The method of administration of a measure, whether patient-, professional- or carer-completed, is a primary concern with this patient population. The advantages and disadvantages of these various methods of recording information have been widely documented and debated.[62,63] In the case of patients receiving palliative care, there is an inherent difficulty using self-completion measures as many patients are too ill to complete them, or die early during care.[64] This results in a lack of information being recorded, leading to potential bias in the results because those patients likely to be experiencing the most problems are less likely to be included in data collection. As an alternative, a final assessment is sometimes completed by a professional, either before or after death. This affects the validity of a measure designed for completion by the patient. Professionally completed measures are frequently used to overcome this particular problem, but by their nature cannot accurately reflect how the patient really feels. Cohen *et al.* argued that the fact that only half of the palliative care population can complete a questionnaire does not mean that health care professionals should not ask those who can rate their quality of life to do so.[65]

The second issue when measuring health outcome for advanced cancer patients is whether a measure includes those domains relevant to palliative care[66] and does not focus on one aspect alone, be it physical symptoms (e.g. the Karnofsky Index)[67] or the existential domain of self-content and well-being. The measures described above address the domains to differing extents, but no single measure covers physical, psychological and spiritual domains in a format that will provide sufficient or reliable information.

The purpose of measuring the quality of life and outcomes of the care of patients is potentially fourfold.[68] One objective is to obtain more detailed information about the patient for clinical monitoring to aid and improve patient care. A second purpose is to audit the care provided, by determining whether standards are being achieved and identify potential areas for improvement. Third, research using outcome measures to compare services, or to compare care before and after the introduction of a service can be of value in assessing the efficacy of a service, and the cost-effectiveness. Finally, analysis of data generated using outcome measures can be used to inform purchasers and thereby secure resources for future services.

Each of the measures described fulfils the objectives to varying degrees, but none of the measures selected successfully meets all of these, and it is questionable whether any such tool can be developed which will meet all the requirements of an 'ideal tool'. However, there is a need to continue researching and developing outcome measures in palliative care that address the concerns outlined above and that could easily be implemented into routine practice. In this way, the provision of palliative care can be monitored and we can continue to strive to obtain the best standards of patient care.

References

1 Wilkin, D., Hallam, L. and Doggett, M.A. (1992) *Measures of Need and Outcome for Primary Health Care.* Oxford: Oxford University Press.

2 Brook, R.H. (1990) Relationship between appropriateness and outcome, in A. Hopkins and D. Bostain (eds) *Measuring the Outcomes of Medical Care*. London: Royal College of Physicians.

3 Bowling, A. (1994) *Measuring Disease: A Review of Disease-specific Quality of Life Measurement Scales*. Buckingham: Open University Press.

4 Calman, K.C. (1984) Quality of life in cancer patients – a hypothesis. *British Journal of Medical Ethics*, 10: 124–7.

5 Higginson, I.J. and McCarthy, M. (1993) Validity of the support team assessment schedule: do staffs' ratings reflect those made by patients or their families? *Palliative Medicine*, 7: 219–28.

6 Ellershaw, J.E., Peat, S.J. and Boys, L.C. (1995) Assessing the effectiveness of a hospital palliative care team. *Palliative Medicine*, 9: 145–52.

7 Bowling, A. (1994) Op. cit.

8 Ibid.

9 Ramsay, M., Winget, C. and Higginson, I. (1995) Review: measures to determine the outcome of community services for people with dementia. *Age and Ageing*, 24 (1): 75–83.

10 Ellershaw, J.E. *et al.* (1995) Op. cit.

11 Morris, J., Suissa, S., Sherwood, S. and Greer, D. (1986) Last days: a study of the quality of life of terminally ill cancer patients. *Journal of Chronic Diseases*, 39: 47–62.

12 Higginson, I. (1993) A community schedule, in I. Higginson (ed.) *Clinical Audit in Palliative Care*. Oxford: Radcliffe Medical Press.

13 MacAdam, D.B. and Smith, M. (1987) An initial assessment of suffering in terminal illness. *Palliative Medicine*, 1: 37–47.

14 Bruera, E., Kuehn, N., Miller, M.J., Selmser, P. and Macmillan, K. (1991) The Edmonton Symptom Assessment System (ESAS): a simple method for the assessment of palliative care patients. *Journal of Palliative Care*, 7 (2): 6–9.

15 Aaronson, N.K., Ahmedzai, S., Bergman, B. *et al.* (1993) The European Organisation for Research and Treatment of Cancer QLQ-C30: a quality-of-life instrument for use in international clinical trials in oncology. *Journal of the National Cancer Institute*, 85: 365–76.

16 Cohen, S.R., Mount, B.M., Strobel, M.G. and Bui, F. (1995) The McGill Quality of Life Questionnaire: a measure of quality of life appropriate for people with advanced disease. A preliminary study of validity and acceptability. *Palliative Medicine*, 9 (3): 207–19.

17 de Haes, J.C.J.M., van Knippenberg, F.C.E. and Neijt, J.P. (1990) Measuring psychological and physical distress in cancer patients: structure and application of the Rotterdam Symptom Checklist. *British Journal of Cancer*, 62: 1034–8.

18 McCorkle, R. and Young, K. (1978) Development of a symptom distress scale. *Cancer Nursing*, 101: 373–8.

19 O'Boyle, C.A., McGee, H. and Joyce, C.R.B. (1994) Quality of life: assessing the individual. *Advances in Medical Sociology*, 5: 159–80.

20 Sterkenburg, C.A. and Woodward, C.A. (1996) A reliability and validity study of the McMaster Quality of Life Scale (MQLS) for a palliative population. *Journal of Palliative Care*, 12 (1): 18–25.

21 Trent Hospice Audit Group (1992) *Palliative Care Core Standards; A Multi-disciplinary Approach*. Trent Hospice Audit, c/o Nightingale Macmillan Continuing Care Unit, Derby.
22 Morris, J. *et al.* (1986) Op. cit.
23 MacAdam, D.B. and Smith, M. (1987) Op. cit.
24 Bruera, E. *et al.* (1991) Op. cit.
25 Aaronson, N.K. *et al.* (1993) Op. cit.
26 Cohen, S.R. *et al.* (1995) Op. cit.
27 de Haes, J.C.J.M. *et al.* (1990) Op. cit.
28 McCorkle, R. and Young, K. (1978) Op. cit.
29 Sterkenburg, C.A. and Woodward, C.A. (1996) Op. cit.
30 Ellershaw, J.E. *et al.* (1995) Op. cit.
31 Higginson, I. (1993) Op. cit.
32 O'Boyle, C.A. *et al.* (1994) Op. cit.
33 Trent Hospice Audit Group (1992) Op. cit.
34 Ellershaw, J.E. *et al.* (1995) Op. cit.
35 MacAdam, D.B. and Smith, M. (1987) Op. cit.
36 Bruera, E. *et al.* (1991) Op. cit.
37 Aaronson, N.K. *et al.* (1993) Op. cit.
38 de Haes, J.C.J.M. *et al.* (1990) Op. cit.
39 McCorkle, R. and Young, K. (1978) Op. cit.
40 Trent Hospice Audit Group (1992) Op. cit.
41 MacAdam, D.B. and Smith, M. (1987) Op. cit.
42 Aaronson, N.K. *et al.* (1993) Op. cit.
43 de Haes, J.C.J.M. *et al.* (1990) Op. cit.
44 O'Boyle, C.A. *et al.* (1994) Op. cit.
45 Sterkenburg, C.A. and Woodward, C.A. (1996) Op. cit.
46 Aaronson, N.K. *et al.* (1993) Op. cit.
47 de Haes, J.C.J.M. *et al.* (1990) Op. cit.
48 MacAdam, D.B. and Smith, M. (1987) Op. cit.
49 Bruera, E. *et al.* (1991) Op. cit.
50 Aaronson, N.K. *et al.* (1993) Op. cit.
51 Morris, J. *et al.* (1986) Op. cit.
52 Cohen, S.R. *et al.* (1995) Op. cit.
53 Sterkenburg, C.A. and Woodward, C.A. (1996) Op. cit.
54 Ellershaw, J.E. *et al.* (1995) Op. cit.
55 Trent Hospice Audit Group (1992) Op. cit.
56 de Haes, J.C.J.M. *et al.* (1990) Op. cit.
57 Rathbone, G.V., Horsley, S. and Goacher, J. (1994) A self-evaluated assessment suitable for seriously ill hospice patients. *Palliative Medicine*, 8 (1): 29–34.
58 Higginson, I. (1993) Op. cit.
59 Higginson, I.J. and McCarthy, M. (1993) Op. cit.
60 McCorkle, R. and Young, K. (1978) Op. cit.
61 O'Boyle, C.A. *et al.* (1994) Op. cit.
62 Bowling, A. (1994) Op. cit.
63 Jenkinson, C. (1994) *Measuring Health and Medical Outcomes*. London: UCL Press.
64 Cohen, S.R. *et al.* (1995) Op. cit.

65 Ibid.
66 Saunders, C.M. (1978) *The Management of Terminal Disease*. London: Edward Arnold.
67 Karnofsky, D.A., Abelmann, W.H., Craver, L.F. *et al.* (1948) The use of nitrogen mustards in the palliative treatment of carcinoma. *Cancer*, I: 634–56.
68 Jenkinson, C. (1994) Op. cit.

Acknowledgements

We would like to thank the NHS Executive Clinical Audit Unit for providing funding for this literature review, which forms part of a larger project developing a new, core measure for use with cancer patients receiving palliative care in a variety of specialist and non-specialist settings. We would also like to thank all the members of the project advisory group for their advice and comments.

Reprinted from *Journal of Public Health Medicine*, J. Hearn and I.J. Higginson, Outcome measures in palliative care for advanced cancer patients: a review, 19(25): 2 193–9, with permission.

PART III

Needs assessment, audit and evaluation

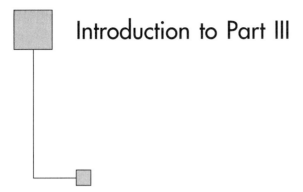

Introduction to Part III

As late as 1973 Saunders and Winner,[1] in reviewing the state of research into the terminal care of cancer patients, were forced to conclude that 'most of the articles which appear in so many of the medical, psychiatric, and sociological journals throughout the world remain descriptive and anecdotal' (p. 21). Since then, partly inspired by major changes in wider health policy,[2] research relating to the planning, delivery and assessment of services to seriously ill and dying people has developed considerably. In Part III of our book such research is highlighted with particular reference to the emerging science of health needs assessment, as well as matters relating to audit and evaluation. In some cases methodological development in these areas has struggled to keep up with the demands of policy makers; but we show here some of the ways in which palliative care researchers have sought to design methods relevant to the requirements of the policy context.

Part III begins with three chapters on needs assessment in palliative care; they can be read in conjunction with a full monograph on the subject, which draws in particular upon epidemiological approaches.[3] The selection here highlights some of the conceptual difficulties in thinking about the assessment of need for palliative care, and also give attention to the overlooked issue of bereavement services. Clark and Malson show how any researcher must be wary of the difficulties involved in defining and measuring need. They suggest that health needs assessment has three principal components: population data, stakeholder perspectives and comparative service data, and indicate some of the methods which might be appropriate to these. Heslop's chapter gives particular attention to the ways in which the views of service users, as key stakeholders, can be incorporated into palliative care needs assessment. This is seen as essentially a collaborative exercise which might make use of such techniques as interviews, surveys, focus groups, or search conferences. Payne and Relf used a survey method to seek information about how palliative care units assess the need for bereavement follow-up. The survey was based around a series of open-ended questions and a process of checking for reliability in coding the responses is described. The chapter is also of interest for its attention to the ways in which service providers themselves make use of particular techniques for assessing the need for bereavement follow-up.

Higginson's chapter in this section of the book provides a useful overview of the development of clinical and organizational audit in palliative care. It also includes details of a range of audit tools which have been in common use in palliative care in recent years. Some of these contain a multidimensional approach to patients' problems, others focus upon the analysis of a single activity or intervention. Most challenging of all are those which focus upon the evaluation of an entire service. Ingleton, Field and Clark shed some light on this in a chapter on 'formative evaluation', in which they put forward a case for the use of qualitative methods. Drawing on the value of a case study design they show how a better understanding of organizational context, achieved through a process of 'triangulation', can lead to evaluation findings which may be both timely and efficacious. Such an approach, which is alert to the complex ordering of activity in a palliative care service, may in turn be complemented by the use of the more structured techniques described by Higginson.

The chapters included in this final section of the book give some idea of the ways in which palliative care researchers have been developing methods to assess need and to measure the impact of services. They show that methodologies must be carefully matched to the research question, that there need be no arbitrary division between qualitative and quantitative approaches, and that despite considerable achievement to date, a great deal of methodological development is required if palliative care policy and practice is to be firmly rooted in the evidence of rigorously conducted research.

Quite how this is to be achieved remains a matter of vigorous debate. Some suggest that the contributions and claims of palliative care will only be established through scrutiny which uses the most searching techniques of randomization.[4] This, therefore, means working out technical solutions to problems of recruitment to studies; consent to randomization; attrition of study subjects; and the timing and character of outcome measures. For others, however, the worth of a palliative care service cannot be adequately evaluated solely on the basis of such research. For example, Keeley[5] poses the question, 'Can we insist on evidence of effectiveness from randomized controlled trials for support services which are of such evident human desirability as to render their deliberate withholding difficult or unethical?' (p. 1147). They would argue that it is morally wrong to deny access to a service simply in the interests of rigorous comparison. In practice, many evaluators of palliative care services and those involved in conducting needs assessments will also be constrained by resource considerations: our studies, to some extent, will only be as good as the funding which is available to support them.

For all these reasons, many studies are likely to inhabit that territory between the descriptive and the analytic. This should not detract from their value. Locally, such work will help to shape strategies and service development – and will be a big step forward from the 'emotional planning' of the early years of the hospice movement. Nationally, studies of this kind are beginning to map out a detailed picture of the current state of the delivery of palliative care. In this context, the multidisciplinary and multimethod approaches favoured by palliative care researchers deserve wider recognition. Despite being at a relatively early stage of its development, palliative care research currently has a great deal to celebrate in its commitment to viewing services in context and in its regular adoption of designs which allow us to look at structure, process and outcome.

References

1 Saunders, C. and Winner, A. (1973) Research into terminal care of cancer patients. *Portfolio for Health 2. The Developing Programme of the DHSS in Health Services Research*. Published for the Nuffield Provincial Hospitals Trust by the Oxford University Press.
2 Clark, D. and Seymour, J. (1999) *Reflections on Palliative Care: Sociological and Policy Perspectives*. Buckingham: Open University Press.
3 Higginson, I. (1997) *Palliative and Terminal Care Health Needs Assessment*. Oxford: Radcliffe Medical Press.
4 McQuay, H. and Moore, A. (1994) Need for rigorous assessment of palliative care. *British Medical Journal*, 309: 1315–16.
5 Keeley, D. (1999) Rigorous assessment of palliative care revisited. *British Medical Journal*, 319: 1447–8.

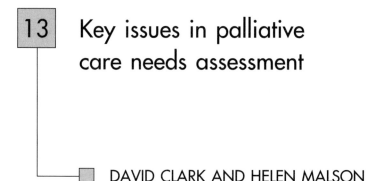

13 Key issues in palliative care needs assessment

DAVID CLARK AND HELEN MALSON

> The very notion of need had proved notoriously difficult to define in ways that could be used in the planning process, and the prospect of arranging a heterogeneous array of needs into an explicit hierarchy of importance for the purpose of deciding service priorities had usually been too daunting even to contemplate.[1]

> Many now view needs assessment as both a political and a technical activity, and are developing needs assessment processes which combine different sources and types of information . . . All are trying to establish needs assessment as a reference point and justification for many decisions.[2]

> . . . the concept of need has always been too imprecise, too complex, too contentious to be a useful target for policy.[3]

These quotations, from observers of the health services in Britain, encapsulate a set of problems which is being unravelled in most of the developed countries of the world. Health care reform is a process which transcends political and geographical boundaries. Underpinning it are several key factors: ageing populations; increased dependency ratios, whereby a dwindling proportion of people who are economically active support the remainder; medical advances and innovations in health care technology; increased consumerism and rising expectations of health care quality and outcome. In the face of these major structural determinants, health services face complex problems associated with the careful management of limited resources. One response to these dilemmas is a growing interest in the merits of market forces *vis-à-vis* regulation and strategic planning. Another, which will be the focus of our discussion here, is the concern to develop health services in relation to the systematic assessment of needs in order to encourage a 'needs-led' health care service. Needs assessment has therefore become the emergent health science of the 1990s. In this chapter we examine the broad aspects of health needs assessment as they relate to palliative care.

Key principles

Pickin and St Leger adopt a thoroughly pragmatic approach to health needs assessment, defining it as 'the process of exploring the relationship between health problems in a community and the resources available to address those problems in order to achieve a desired outcome'.[4] The effectiveness of such an assessment would therefore depend upon how needs are defined and the ways in which they are measured.

There are of course a number of conceptual difficulties surrounding the definition of need itself, which focus on how broadly need should be perceived for policy purposes. In the UK context of purchasing for health or social care, need is defined narrowly as the population's ability to benefit from specific services relating to specific problems.[5,6] This definition has two key dimensions. Need is inextricably linked first with service provision, and secondly with the ability to *benefit* from health or social care. It has been pointed out however that *need* does not necessarily equate with *demand*, which may simply reflect historical circumstances or even the interests and preferences of particular local clinicians.[7] At the same time *supply* may not be well matched to need. Within this functional conception of need, therefore, the ability of the population to benefit from an intervention depends on two things: the incidence and prevalence of a particular condition and the effectiveness of the services available to deal with it.

The definition thus embodies a focus on the outcomes of care interventions: if purchasing authorities are to improve health and social well-being, then their aim must be to secure proven, effective provision. The benefit must also be produced at reasonable risk and acceptable cost if it is to be regarded as appropriate for making changes in current provision. In a policy context, then, needs are increasingly couched in the language of priorities, addressing questions such as who is to have first claim on limited resources, and who is to judge that claim. From this perspective needs are relative and often have to be traded off against each other, given limited resources.[8] The vulnerability of palliative care services in such a policy context is obvious, especially when compared to the demands of the more technological aspects of curative medicine.

The functional conception of need is worrying in other ways. By assuming that needs only exist where there are services which might meet them, we embark on a dangerous teleology which is calculated to overlook needs that are difficult to conceptualize, identify or respond to. In palliative care, needs associated with psychological or spiritual suffering might come into this category, but so too might complex physical symptoms, or the social needs of those who are caring for the sick person. Indeed, we might argue that one of the crucial successes of hospice and palliative care has been its ability to identify problems and needs which generic services have overlooked, ignored or found too difficult. Palliative care has created a response to these needs which improves well-being and quality of life at a variety of levels.

For these reasons health needs assessment must be inclusive in its approach and constructed in ways which allow previously unidentified or unanticipated needs to be defined. This has a bearing in turn on research design and choice of methodologies. To be successful, health needs assessment must go beyond approaches rooted in patient/user satisfaction or quality assurance, important elements though these are. The focus should rather be on *communities* and *individuals* with collective and personal expressions of need. Inevitably, these expressions may at times be weakly articulated or vaguely defined; the task of needs assessment however is to give some structure and clarity to these expressions.

Components and methods

Seen in this way, health needs assessment has three principal components (Figure 13.1).

Population data

An analysis of epidemiological and demographic data forms the first key dimension of any assessment of health need. This in a sense is the familiar territory of public health planning. In the palliative care context it will include the incidence and prevalence of conditions such as cancer, coronary heart disease, and cerebrovascular disease, taking into account local and regional variations. In most Western countries the increasing proportion of older people in the population, coupled with the higher prevalence of both cancer and a number of chronic conditions, form an important set of interrelated issues.[9,10]

The health needs of a local population will also reflect its socioeconomic, cultural and ethnic character.[11-13] Variations and patterns in *where* people die should also be taken into account. In the West it has become common for a high proportion of people to die in hospital; to what extent does this meet their needs and those of their carers? It has also been suggested that where people die may relate to underlying structural factors, such as poverty and social deprivation.[14] All of these will be important epidemiological and demographic dimensions to be taken into account in a palliative care needs assessment. Attention to non-malignant conditions will also be of

Figure 13.1   Components of health needs assessment

Population data	Stakeholder perspectives	Comparative data
• Epidemiological • Demographic	• Users (patients and informal carers) • Providers • Community groups • Purchasers and planners	• Costs • Outputs • Outcomes

importance, as palliative care attempts to move beyond its traditional focus on cancer.[15]

Stakeholder perspectives

The second key dimension of palliative care needs assessment is more qualitative in orientation. This is a potentially challenging area in which the perspectives of key stakeholders are sought and interrelationships between them explored. Key stakeholders will include: service users (patients and informal carers); providers (of health and social care); local community groups (with or without a specialist interest in health), as well as those charged with responsibilities for the funding, organization and planning of services.

Viewed in this way, health needs assessment becomes a political process, as inevitably the viewpoints of different individuals and groups will not always coincide and may at times conflict with one another. This aspect of needs assessment is perhaps best aided at the collective level by the skills of the sociologist or anthropologist, and at the individual level by psychological approaches. The aim of these analyses will be to generate a detailed picture of community health needs, focusing on the views of users (actual or potential), purchasers and providers of services. Palliative care has a good deal to learn here from the use of community development methodologies, where users and local people are not merely seen as 'consumers' of services, but as key stakeholders in how needs assessments are conducted as well as agents in the strategic planning and purchasing processes.[16,17] Several research methods lend themselves to this aspect of health needs assessment: interviews, focus groups, surveys, participant observation, rapid appraisal.

Comparative data

The third strand in the needs assessment framework focuses less on the quantification or elucidation of need and more on how needs, as currently perceived, are being met. In other words, this part of the process is concerned with the costs, outputs and outcomes of services, in particular when examined comparatively across districts and regions.[18] This aspect of health needs assessment therefore draws on skills in health technology assessment and in health economics. Equity is an important consideration here, since access to palliative care services may vary with the local availability of hospital and hospice in-patient care, domiciliary care, respite and day care, and bereavement services. There is still remarkably little systematic evidence on the comparative costs and volumes associated with these services and still less on their effectiveness.[19]

Conclusions: the promise of palliative care needs assessment

Health needs assessment is a newly developing approach to planning care. It is based on the rational premise that a comprehensive assessment of need should precede the implementation of services, allowing these to be more sensitively tailored to local conditions and concerns. In palliative care where what might be called *emotional planning* has often predominated over more systematic approaches, the importance of careful assessment of needs is of major importance. A number of difficulties however will continue to challenge those involved in palliative care needs assessment:

- We must become clearer on how complex psychosocial, spiritual and physical needs can be described and conceptualized, allowing unexpressed needs and the needs of disadvantaged groups to be more fully articulated.
- We must develop multidisciplinary and innovative methodologies to allow us to identify and analyse needs.
- We must recognize that the language of need takes us on to the problem of priorities: where resources are limited, whose palliative care needs will predominate?

Health needs assessment in palliative care requires considerable attention if it is to be useful in improving services.

References

1 Butler, J. (1993) *Patients, Policies and Politics*. Buckingham: Open University Press, pp. 74–5.
2 Ovretveit, J. (1995) *Purchasing for Health*. Buckingham: Open University Press, p. 14.
3 Bradshaw, J. (1994) The conceptualisation and measurement of need: a social policy perspective, in J. Popay and G. Williams (eds) *Researching the People's Health*. London: Routledge, p. 45.
4 Pickin, C. and St Leger, S. (1993) *Assessing Health Need Using the Life Cycle Framework*. Buckingham: Open University Press, p. 6.

5 National Health Service Management Executive (1991) *Moving Forward: Needs, Services and Contracts*. London: NHSME.

6 National Health Service Management Executive (1991) *Assessing Health Care Needs: A DHA Project Discussion Paper*. London: NHSME.

7 Stevens, A. and Gabbay, J. (1991) Needs assessment needs assessment. *Health Trends*, 23: 20–3.

8 Williams, A. (1992) Priorities – not needs, in A. Corden, G. Robertson and K. Tolley (eds) *Meeting Needs*. Aldershot: Avebury.

9 Higginson, I. and Victor, C. (1994) Needs assessment for older people. *Journal of the Royal Society of Medicine of London*, 87: 471–3.

10 Yancik, R. and Ries, L.A. (1994) Cancer in older persons: magnitude of the problem – how do we apply what we know? *Cancer*, 74 (7 Supplement): 1995–2003.

11 Black, D. (1982) Inequalities in Health: The Black Report. London: Penguin.

12 Robertson, N.L. (1994) Breast cancer screening in older black women. *Cancer*, 74 (7 Supplement): 2034–40.

13 Eames, M., Ben-Shlomo, Y. and Marmot, M.G. (1993) Social deprivation and premature mortality: regional comparison across England. *British Medical Journal*, 307: 1097–102.

14 Higginson, I., Webb, D. and Lessof, L. (1994) Reducing hospital beds for patients with advanced cancer. [Letter] *Lancet*, 844: 409.

15 Standing Medical Advisory Committee and Standing Nursing and Midwifery Advisory Committee (1992) *The Principles and Provision of Palliative Care*. London: HMSO.

16 Ong, B.N. and Humphris, G. (1994) Rapid appraisal methodologies, in J. Popay and G. Williams (eds) (1994) *Researching the People's Health*. London: Routledge.

17 National Health Service Management Executive (1992) *Local Voices: The Views of Local People in Purchasing for Health*. Leeds: NHSME.

18 Neale, B., Clark, D. and Heather, H. (1993) *Purchasing Palliative Care: A Review of the Policy and Research Literature*, Occasional Paper 11. Sheffield: Trent Palliative Care Centre.

19 Small, N., Ashworth, A., Coyle, D. *et al.* (1995) *Standard Setting, Cost and Effectiveness in Palliative Care Services*. London: Department of Health.

Acknowledgement

Clark, D. and Malson, H. (1995) Key issues in palliative care needs assessment, *Progress in Palliative Care*, 3: 53–5, reprinted with permission of Leeds Medical Information.

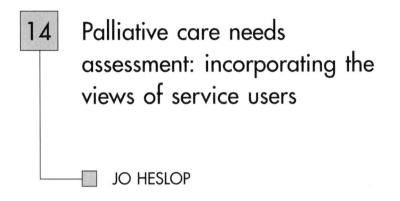

14 Palliative care needs assessment: incorporating the views of service users

JO HESLOP

Health Authorities which are serious about establishing needs cannot just do research on communities but have to do it with communities.[1]

Health needs assessment, the 'emergent health science of the 1990s',[2] has been described by Clark and Malson as having three principal components: population data, stakeholder perspectives and comparative data.[3] Service users (both patients and informal carers) and community groups (who may or may not have a particular involvement in health services) are to be found alongside purchasers, providers and planners in the group described as stakeholders. Having recognized the role of service users in health needs assessment, at what point are they to be included? There are two contrasting approaches to the effective involvement of service users. The first has been to see patients as consumers, who have the right to choose and to comment upon the services which they receive. Their views are commonly sought by such means as questionnaires and surveys designed to elicit information about their levels of satisfaction with completed proposals or existing services. The problem with this approach is that consultation occurs at a stage when it is difficult for a valuable contribution to be made – decisions about service provision have already been taken. The second approach is to see service users as partners in services, involved in the design, delivery and evaluation of services.[4] This approach, which has been developed in the UK in response to the changes brought about by the NHS and Community Care Act,[5] requires a recognition of the need to involve service users at an early stage, before plans have taken shape. 'Plans may not always be written in tablets of stone but they do have a habit of resisting amendment once

Figure 14.1 The purchasing cycle

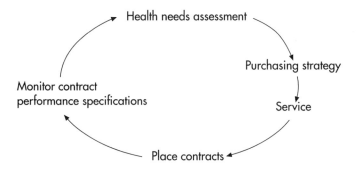

they have been drafted.'[6] Of course many health care services are already well established: the phenomenon which is new is that of the purchasing cycle (Figure 14.1).[7]

The systematic inclusion of needs assessment, bringing together 'hard' data drawn from available statistics and 'soft' data gleaned from the views of local people, within the purchasing cycle should lead to a service which is responsive to the concerns of the people for whom it is provided. This being said, how are the views of service users, either actual or potential, to be elicited? Are there any factors particular to palliative care which inform the ways in which information about needs is sought? A number of methods are useful in seeking information, each of which should be used with a considerable degree of sensitivity. People who are receiving palliative care, either as patients or as carers, are facing many difficulties and sorrows and are therefore potentially very vulnerable. Differing degrees of knowledge and understanding about the situation in which they find themselves, and varying ability to discuss it, may well be in evidence: between one patient and another; between patient and carer and even, at different times, within one patient. An awareness of potentially upsetting topics should also be borne in mind when working with those with no apparent current contact with palliative care, as painful memories of past bereavements may be brought to the surface.

The majority of health service research projects are carried out with the consent of the local medical ethics committee, a process which provides safeguards for those patients who are involved in the research. There must also be ethical considerations in respect of those for whom an application to the medical ethics committee is not required. These are neatly summarized by Sykes *et al.* as a number of obligations to those who take part in the research, namely that they should not be misled about the purpose or nature of the research in order to encourage their participation; that assurances of confidentiality are honoured, and that they should not be damaged in any way by taking part.[8]

Individual interviews

The use of in-depth interviews, conducted by skilled professionals, is one of the most important research tools that can be called into play when working with palliative care patients and their informal carers. It is a method which can take into account the vulnerability of the interviewee while giving her or him the opportunity to contribute to the research and thus to the development of palliative care services.[9] Setting up such interviews is a process which is not, however, without its difficulties,[10] and, where they have been attempted, randomized trials involving palliative care patients have been shown to be problematic, chiefly due to difficulties in recruitment and early deaths of patients.[11] Notwithstanding the practical problems involved in the organization of individual interviews with palliative care patients and their carers, interviews can provide a valuable opportunity for those with a very real understanding of palliative care needs to give a direct account of what they want from services. The use of semi-structured interview schedules helps to give direction to the interview while not precluding the identification of new or previously unidentified issues of concern. One consequence of separate interviewing of patients and carers may be that different perceptions of need, or even direct conflict in views about services, may be revealed, a factor which should be recognized when data is being analysed.

The survey

Surveys, while they may lack the richness of detail to be gleaned from in-depth interviews, provide a way of acquiring information which contributes to the formation of 'the big picture'. Surveys can be aimed at individuals or groups, such as self-help and support groups or community organizations, or at people linked by a common factor, such as a particular diagnosis, and may take the form of interviews, both face-to-face and by telephone, and through the use of postal questionnaires.[12-14] Target populations may be selected by those carrying out the research[15] or they may self-select by, for example, responding to a media appeal to take part in the project.[16] This type of research, where there may be little direct contact with a skilled interviewer, raises the question of how potentially vulnerable respondents may be protected. Safeguards such as the provision of information about local support groups or relevant helpline telephone numbers can be of value.

The focus group

The focus group has been used as a way of assessing public perception of a wide range of health service issues. Groups of local people, who may be drawn at random from the general population or who may represent a particular group, have been brought together to discuss a variety of topics.[17] The focus group can also be used as a method for comparing the perspectives of different but related groups of people about the same topic.[18] This is a method of inquiry which can be of value in palliative care needs assessment. Members of specialist groups which have an interest in palliative care issues, for instance self-help groups run by people with a specific health problem such as multiple sclerosis or cancer, or groups who offer bereavement support, can offer valuable insights. Members of community groups with no particular health care remit, but nevertheless with valuable comment to offer, can also be invited to meet to discuss palliative care needs.

The search conference

The aim of the search conference is to 'encourage mutual understanding and coordinated action among different groups of people who share a common concern about a particular issue or set of issues, but who approach it from different perspectives'.[19] The search process which drives the conference helps people to work in a way which acknowledges their differences, with the aim of developing an understanding of each other's needs. In such a forum it may be possible to bring together patients and their carers for joint discussion. Clearly this will not be a suitable method for those who are very near to the end of their lives, but it may be a valuable method of examining the needs of those with chronic and debilitating life-threatening illnesses, who often feel that their needs are neglected in favour of those with malignant disease, and would aid the planning of palliative care services for this group of people.[20,21]

Rapid appraisal

Participatory rapid appraisal has been developed as a method which aims to gain an understanding of a community's own perspectives on its own principal needs.[22] Rapid appraisal offers information about the nature of particular problems rather than the number of people affected by them. A community is defined as a social rather than a geographic entity and therefore an understanding of that community must be built up through various perspectives which are present within the community. Information is gathered from selected people, known as 'key informants', who have a particular knowledge about the community. These key informants can be drawn from the following groups: professionals, such as general practitioners, teachers, social workers and nurses; leaders of local groups which could include local councillors and community group leaders; people who could be described as being social focal points, for example, shopkeepers and publicans.[23] As its name implies, rapid appraisal is a method which is designed to be undertaken with greater speed than more conventional methods of analysis. A method which employs a multidisciplinary and semi-structured approach, and which allows for a degree of flexibility, lends itself to use in the field of palliative care.

Conclusions

It is some twenty-five years [in 1995] since the notion of service user participation was first mooted in the UK and it is now firmly on the policy agenda. Systematic needs assessment is, however, a new and challenging concept, and the difficulties of actively involving patients who are facing death and their informal carers must not be underestimated. At a time of scarce resources there is also the problem of raising expectations which may be worked towards but not, at least in the short term, met.

- We must foster a culture in which service users have a genuine place in needs assessment and in the continuing cycle of purchasing and evaluating palliative care services.
- We must strive to develop sensitive, flexible and efficient ways of working together with palliative care service users in order to define their needs.
- We must develop a relationship with palliative care service users in order to ensure a continuing dialogue between service providers and service users.

Health care needs assessment is a new and challenging process and there is much work to be done to ensure its successful development. Palliative care, with its tradition of innovation in areas such as holistic care and the multidisciplinary team approach, is well placed to meet the challenge.

References

1 Ong, B.N. and Humphris, G. (1990) Partners in need. *Health Service Journal*, 100: 1002–3.
2 Clark, D. and Malson, H. (1995) Key issues in palliative care needs assessment. *Progress in Palliative Care*, 3 (2): 53.
3 Ibid.
4 Gleave, R. and Peck, E. (1992) *Commissioning Priority Services*. Bristol: NHS Training Directorate.
5 *NHS and Community Care Act* (1990) London: HMSO.
6 Wertheimer, A. (ed.) (1991) *A Chance to Speak Out: Consulting Service Users and Carers about Community Care*. London: King's Fund Centre, p. viii.

 7 Neale, B., Clark, D. and Heather, P. (1993) *Purchasing Palliative Care: A Review of the Policy and Research Literature*, Occasional Paper 11. Sheffield: Trent Palliative Care Centre.
 8 Sykes, W., Collins, M., Hunter, J., Popay, J. and Williams, G. (1992) *Listening to Local Voices: A Guide to Research Methods, Vol. 3*. Leeds: Nuffield Institute for Health Services Studies, University of Leeds and the Public Health Research and Resource Centre, Salford.
 9 Higginson, I., Wade, W. and McCarthy, M. (1990) Palliative care: views of patients and their families. *British Medical Journal*, 301: 277–81.
10 Clark, D., Heslop, J. and Malson, H. (1996) *As Much Help as Possible: Assessing Palliative Care Needs in Southern Derbyshire*, Occasional Paper 19. Sheffield: Trent Palliative Care Centre.
11 McWhinney, I.R., Bass, M.J. and Donner, A. (1994) Evaluation of a palliative care service: problems and pitfalls. *British Medical Journal*, 309: 1340–2.
12 Field, D., Dand, P., Ahmedzai, S. and Biswas, B. (1996) Care and information received by lay carers of terminally ill patients at the Leicestershire Hospice. *Palliative Medicine*, 6: 237–45.
13 Spiller, J. and Alexander, D. (1993) Domiciliary care: a comparison of the views of terminally ill patients and their family caregivers. *Palliative Medicine*, 7: 109–15.
14 Nicholas, A. and Frankenberg, R. (1992) *Towards a Strategy for Palliative Care: A Needs Assessment for Nottingham Health Department of Public Health*. Nottingham: Nottinghan Health.
15 Kurti, L. (1993) *Palliative Care in Non-malignant Disease: The Carer's Perspective*. Derby: Derbyshire Medical Advisory Group and University of Nottingham.
16 McWhinney, I.R. *et al.* (1994) Op. cit.
17 National Health Service Management Executive (1992) *Local Voices: The Views of Local People in Purchasing for Health*. Leeds: NHS Management Executive.
18 Kahn, S., Houts, P. and Harding, S. (1992) Quality of life and patients with cancer: a comparative study of patient versus physician perceptions and its implications for cancer education. *Journal of Cancer Education*, 7: 241–9.
19 Wertheimer, A. (ed.) (1991) Op. cit., p. 4.
20 Clark, D. and Malson, H. (1995) Op. cit.
21 Spiller, J. and Alexander, D. (1993) Op. cit.
22 Murray, S.A., Tapson, J., Turnbull, L., McCallum, J. and Little, A. (1994) Listening to local voices: adapting rapid appraisal to assess health and social needs in general practice. *British Medical Journal*, 308: 698–700.
23 Ong, B.N. (1993) *The Practice of Health Services Research*. London: Chapman Hall.

Acknowledgement

Heslop, J. (1995) Palliative care needs assessment: incorporating the views of service users, *Progress in Palliative Care*, 3: 135–7, reprinted with permission of Leeds Medical Information.

15 The assessment of need for bereavement follow-up in palliative and hospice care

SHEILA PAYNE AND MARILYN RELF

Introduction

The emphasis placed on family-centred care means that continuing support after a patient's death is, logically, an integral component of palliative care. Despite recommendations that bereavement follow-up should be available[1,2] no clear rationale for the delivery of services has developed.[3] The range of services provided includes group work, one-to-one counselling, telephone contact, social activities, mutual support groups and written information about grief and bereavement.[4] There is a lack of general agreement, however, about what bereavement care should involve[5] and there have been few attempts to evaluate services.

The only strategy to be systematically scrutinized is the provision of one-to-one support or bereavement counselling. This strategy has only been found to be effective when targeted using risk factors associated with poor outcome.[6,7] Risk factors are characteristics of bereaved people or features of their circumstances that increase vulnerability and slow down adjustment[8] and have been identified by a number of studies.[9,10] Studies of support offered to unselected bereaved people have found no benefit.[11] Indeed, it has been suggested that offering support to people who have adequate internal and external resources can undermine coping and be detrimental rather than helpful.[12] Parkes argues that palliative care is in a unique position to offer preventative support, that assessment of need should be routine and that it promotes the efficient utilization of resources.[13] At St Christopher's Hospice he introduced a questionnaire, completed by nursing staff, that provided a numerical score as a measure of risk. Decisions about follow-up were based on this score.[14]

Two studies have reported on the use of risk indexes and checklists to assess need and to target bereavement services. In the USA, Lattanzi-Licht[15] surveyed 268 hospices and found that, while services were very diverse, 88 per cent made telephone calls after a death and 83 per cent visited the bereaved. Over half (58 per cent) used formal methods of risk assessment. In Australia, Gibson and Graham[16] surveyed 122 hospices and found that just over half provided bereavement support and that one-third used formal risk assessment.

A recent survey by Wilkes[17] illustrated the range of bereavement services provided by palliative care units in this country, but revealed little about the way in which the needs of bereaved people are assessed or how decisions are made about the allocation of services.

The aims of this present study were:

1 To assess the extent and prevalence of bereavement support services provided by palliative care units in the UK.
2 To explore the methods used to allocate bereavement support services.

Method

A postal questionnaire survey was conducted in the summer of 1992. A total of 397 questionnaires were posted to palliative care units, including in-patient units, hospital support teams and Macmillan services, identified from the *Directory of Hospice Services in the UK and Ireland 1992*;[18] single-handed Macmillan nurses were excluded. A total of 187 responses were returned, a response rate of 47 per cent. One questionnaire could not be coded and the results are based on 186 replies. The questionnaires were separately and independently rated by an impartial research assistant and one of the authors (SP). It was considered desirable to have one rater who was not involved in the conception and design of the study, to ensure that potential biases resulting from the authors' involvement with bereavement research and services would not influence the results.

Measures

A questionnaire was developed based on that used by Gibson and Graham.[19] Ten open-ended questions covered the following topics: type of bereavement follow-up service, type of risk assessment used, profession of assessor, and evaluation of current assessment method. In addition, we asked for details of the post held by the person completing the survey. Respondents were also asked to enclose examples of any standardized bereavement risk assessment tools currently in use in their unit. Reply paid envelopes were enclosed and a covering letter introduced the questionnaire and informed respondents that this was part of a research project.

Table 15.1   Provision of bereavement follow-up

	n	%
Bereavement follow-up	156	84
Intend to provide follow-up	13	7
No bereavement follow-up	14	7
Not codable	3	2
Totals	186	100

Results

One hundred and eighty-six questionnaires were submitted to content analysis. A strict coding structure was developed. Inter-rater reliability reached an acceptable level of $r = 0.89$ and any difficulties in coding were resolved by discussion. We were unable to code one question: 'When is the assessment of need completed in relation to the bereavement?' because this was ambiguous. Some interpreted it to mean, 'When did they make the assessment?' and others answered it in relation to when they terminated contact with bereaved people. The majority of questionnaires, 120 (65 per cent) were completed by nurses, 31 (17 per cent) by social workers, 12 (6 per cent) by bereavement coordinators and 23 (12 per cent) by others.

Type of service

Table 15.1 shows the extent of services provided; 156 respondents (84 per cent) were providing some type of bereavement follow-up and a further 13 (17 per cent) expressed their intention to develop their services. Those not offering support were predominantly hospital support teams. The impression was gained that this is a period of transition in the provision of bereavement support; 34 units reported that their services were under review, 22 units were involved in establishing new services, and 22 units were hoping to extent their existing services. We received 20 requests for help or information.

Table 15.2 shows the range of strategies of bereavement support. This includes 30 units which made onward referrals to other agencies such as Cruse, the national organization for the widowed and bereaved.

Allocation of bereavement services

The majority of units, 132 (71 per cent), either made no assessment or used only informal assessment procedures. Formal assessment was defined as a written form such as an index, questionnaire or checklist. Respondents were specifically asked if they used a standardized questionnaire or measure.

Table 15.2   Strategies of bereavement follow-up offered

Strategy	n	%
Telephone contact	23	12
Personal visits	35	19
Group sessions/social meetings	40	22
Onward referral	30	16
Not known/no response	58	31
Total	186	100

It was found that only 48 (26 per cent) were using formal tools, although a further 15 (8 per cent) reported that they intended to do so in the future. Standardized measures were completed by nurses in 41 units (85 per cent), by the clinical team in six units (12 per cent); in one unit it was completed by the bereavement service coordinator. The assessment of need is thus predominantly regarded as being within the nurse's role.

The criteria used to allocate services was examined in the 125 units who provided bereavement follow-up but who did not make formal assessments. Fifty-eight units (46 per cent) reported basing their decisions on discussions amongst the professionals involved, or deciding on 'gut feelings'. The next largest group, 39 (32 per cent), provided follow-up to everyone by visiting or telephoning. Finally, 11 units (9 per cent) reported on relying on people to self-refer; they might provide information on available services but then left it to individuals to opt into the services they required.

Evaluation of current methods of assessment

Respondents were asked to describe the advantages of their current assessment methods. They could mention more than one aspect. The responses were grouped into five categories: flexibility, objectivity, open to all, convenience, and non-intrusiveness. Responses were compared between those using formal and informal assessments. Units using formal assessments claimed that objectivity was the main advantage while those using informal assessments liked the flexibility, convenience and apparent openness of their current approaches (Table 15.3).

Respondents were asked to describe any problems they were having with their assessment methods. They could mention as many problems as they wished. Responses were grouped into three categories: failure to identify the right people in need of support, limited resources for bereavement follow-up, and problems with the assessment method itself. Units using formal risk assessment were compared with those that were not (Table 15.4). Both groups expressed dissatisfaction with their current assessment techniques.

Table 15.3   Advantages of current assessment methods

Assessment	Flexible	Objective	Openness	Convenience	Non-intrusiveness
Formal (*n* = 48)	9	23	9	3	1
Informal (*n* = 125)	33	0	18	11	3

Table 15.4   Disadvantages of current assessment methods

Assessment	Not targeting right people	Limited resources	Assessment problems
Formal (*n* = 48)	3	14	20
Informal (*n* = 125)	17	38	21

Those using informal assessments reported more problems, however, with concerns focusing on limited resources and anxieties about whether or not they were correctly identifying people in need of support.

Analysis of standardized risk assessment measures

Forty-two assessment forms were received from the 48 units using formal methods. The measures were submitted to content analysis.

Who was assessed?

Thirty-seven measures focused assessment on one individual, but of these 15 had some provision for including an assessment of the needs of other family members. Only five forms were designed to assess more than one person.

When were assessments made?

In the majority of cases, 39 (81 per cent), assessment was made either immediately after or within one week of the death; only three forms included some aspect of assessment done prior to the death.

Format of measures

The most popular format was open-ended questioning (*n* = 24), followed by checklists (*n* = 14) and yes/no questions (*n* = 11). Only four used rating scales, and just three were weighted. One measure might incorporate a number of these response modes.

Table 15.5 Factors most frequently assessed in 42 bereavement risk assessment forms

Factors	n	%
Social	202	41
Personal	126	25
Circumstantial	170	34
Total	498	100

Content of measures

The content of the forms was categorized into three areas: circumstantial factors at or near the time of death, personal factors, and social factors (Table 15.5). Circumstantial and social factors were more frequently assessed than personal factors.

Each of these broad categories was made up of 13 subcategories, with a total of 39 separate subcategories being utilized. Table 15.6 shows only those subcategories used by five or more assessment forms.

Discussion

Clearly, bereavement support is considered to be an important part of palliative care, and most respondents were aware of the concept of risk assessment. Asking for help requires courage at a time when the bereaved person may be too depressed and insecure to take the initiative;[20,21] it was encouraging that few units were reliant on self-referral alone.

The majority of units were assessing the need for bereavement support. It was surprising, given Parkes's leading role in the field, that only one-quarter were using formal procedures. This proportion was greater than that reported by the Australian survey,[22] but was much lower than that reported by Lattanzi-Licht in the USA.[23] The question of why so few palliative care services are using formal risk assessment tools is particularly pertinent, given the current climate of financial restraint and the need to justify the use of resources.

Many respondents sent long letters with the returned questionnaires. Overall, our impression was that they were under a great deal of pressure from heavy workloads in combination with limited resources; this finding echoes the work of Lattanzi-Licht in the USA,[24] who reported that services suffered from insufficient staff time, and a lack of personnel and funding.

In our survey, limited resources were described as the major disadvantage associated with informal assessment and were a particular problem for

Table 15.6   Factors identified in formal assessment measures

Subcategory	n
Circumstantial	
Previous loss	31
Dependants	30
Financial position	26
Concurrent life crises	20
Difficult death	17
Housing situation	16
Sudden death	14
Body image issues	10
Death of a child	6
Personal	
Previous mental health	20
Anxiety	14
Anger	14
Emotional symptoms	13
Guilt	12
Suicide risk	11
Physical health	9
Grief	8
Drug use	7
Alcohol	7
Personality	6
Depression	5
Social	
Family characteristics	33
Family support	29
Social support	24
Emotional dependence on deceased	23
Absence or presence at death	20
Awareness of diagnosis	16
Family tree	14
Spiritual support	12
Difficulty in making decisions	10
Marital relationship	8
Self-care difficulties	7
Member of caring profession	6

community-based home care and Macmillan nurses. Using standardized measures involves training staff in the use of risk factors, the routine completion of assessment forms, discussion and reflection. Moreover, it implies that experienced bereavement support personnel, professional or volunteer, will be available to provide support to those identified as being in need. The reliance on informal assessment may simply reflect the lack of time available for systematic bereavement care. Unfortunately it was not possible for us to test this hypothesis by correlating methods of risk assessment with support strategies.

Respondents liked the flexibility and convenience of informal assessment, suggesting that it fits more easily into the workload and is less time-consuming. Experience and instinct should not be denigrated; Parkes found that nurses' intuitive feelings were the best predictors of outcome.[25] However, reliance on experience raises a number of issues. How do we ensure that criteria are being used consistently? How can experience be passed on? In what ways can assessors check that personal likes, dislikes and prejudices are not influencing their decisions? Those using formal measures felt that their decisions were objective, whereas those drawing on their experience were anxious about whether they were identifying the right people. One advantage of using a risk index is that it enables subjective judgements to be scrutinized.

Respondents using formal methods expressed concerns with assessment tools. As in the Australian and American surveys, the majority of measures sent to us derived from Parkes's risk index. Two studies have examined the use of this index, reporting only limited support for its reliability. Beckwick et al.[26] found that the index was only predictive of outcome at three months after bereavement but not at one, six or twelve months. Levy et al.[27] examined the internal validity of the index as well as its reliability. They found that the internal consistency was low (Cronbach's alpha = 0.50) and concluded that it could not be relied upon as a predictor of outcome and that the reasons for this lay within the instrument itself. Further examination of the principal components revealed that nurses' judgement of a person's ability to cope was the most reliable predictor of outcome. They argued that the instrument was not tapping sufficiently the clinical judgement of staff and suggested a number of ways in which it could be improved. The extensive work on risk factors could provide the basis for revision, or a new tool could be generated directly from the clinical experience of nurses. This study[28] provides reassurance for those using informal methods of assessment but the authors stress that, if human judgement is to be used, attempts to improve it must also be taken and training must be provided. Although nurses' coping predictions correlated with outcome measures, the levels of statistical significance were not high.

It is clear that assessment lies within the nurse's role. Risk assessment is rooted in the belief that nurses will have known the family over a period of time before the crisis of the death. Demographic data on patients in the hospice in which one of the authors works reveals a decline in recent years in both overall duration of contact with patients and the amount of time spent as in-patients.[29] This means that nurses' knowledge of key carers may be limited and be less than that envisaged by Parkes. This moves the nurse into the arena of seeking additional information from key carers (for example about their mental health), which some feel is intrusive. The training and support needs of nurses involved in any form of risk assessment must be recognized. The role carries with it the responsibility of possibly denying support to those in need. Indeed this fear was frequently expressed as a justification for offering support to all.

Risk assessment was conceived as a way of targeting one-to-one bereavement support and not as a way of screening access to other aspects of a bereavement service such as social evenings. This concept was not always understood by respondents and some felt that a low-risk categorization meant that no support should be offered. There are a number of ways in which hospice care attempts to meet the diverse needs of the bereaved.[30] Some strategies, such as providing written information about grief, will be useful to all, but only a minority are likely to need long-term one-to-one support.

The desire to offer support to everyone was clearly related to concerns about correct assessment, but the needs of staff should also be recognized. Key carers may have developed a great deal of trust in the staff and shared deeply personal concerns prior to the patient's death. In these circumstances it can be very difficult to say goodbye to newly bereaved people, no matter how resourceful they are. Knowing that people are likely to cope does not remove the desire to want to stay involved just to be sure.

There is insufficient space in this chapter to present a thorough discussion of the variables included in the tools forwarded to us. Indeed we did not set out to examine the tools themselves, but to comment on their use. It was striking, however, that most were framed in terms of pathology rather than resilience, and that measures of coping ability tended to be indirectly rather than directly assessed.

The response rate was disappointing. A number of respondents commented that it was unfortunate that this study was carried out so soon after Wilkes's[31] survey of hospice bereavement services, even though there was minimal overlap. Wilkes's response rate (56 per cent) was also rather low, suggesting that other factors may have been present.

Conclusion

Bereavement follow-up is recognized as part of palliative care, but pressure of work, lack of time and resources are limiting factors. Risk assessment is held to be a way of ensuring that follow-up is directed toward vulnerable people. This study revealed that the majority of palliative care units do assess risk and that this is undertaken by nurses. Most relied on experience rather than standardized measures to target support. Informal assessment was regarded as more flexible and convenient but was associated with more problems. Concerns were expressed about the accuracy of judgements, and units using informal methods were less likely to have sufficient resources to provide ongoing support. Those using standardized measures liked their objectivity but had concerns about the tools they were using. There is a need for further study of how we can improve the use of risk factors to identify bereaved people in need of additional intervention. Standardized tools should be improved and designed in collaboration with nurse assessors, and resourcefulness and coping abilities should be considered alongside the likely occurrence of complications. The training needs of nurses assessing risk must be addressed to ensure that clinical criteria are used thoughtfully and consistently.

Finally, there is a need for wider discussion of the purpose and scope of bereavement services in palliative care. Without agreement about what constitutes good practice it will be difficult to secure adequate resources to offer systematic follow-up.

References

1 Wilkes, E. (1980) *Report of the Working Group on Terminal Care.* London: Standing Medical Advisory Committee, DHSS.
2 National Association of Health Authorities and Trusts (1991) *Care of People with Terminal Illness.* Report by a Joint Advisory Group. Birmingham: NAHAT.
3 Faulkner, A. (1993) Developments in bereavement services, in D. Clark (ed.) *The Future for Palliative Care: Issues of Policy and Practice.* Buckingham: Open University Press.
4 Wilkes, E. (1993) Characteristics of hospice bereavement services. *Journal of Cancer Care,* 2: 183–9.
5 Faulkner, A. (1993) Op. cit.
6 Raphael, B. (1977) Preventive intervention with the recently bereaved. *Archives of General Psychiatry,* 34: 1450–4.
7 Parkes, C.M. (1981) Evaluation of a bereavement service. *Journal of Preventive Psychiatry,* 1: 179–88.
8 Stroebe, M.S. and Stroebe, W. (1993) Determinants of adjustment to bereavement in younger widows and widowers, in M.S. Stroebe, W. Stroebe and R.O. Hansson (eds) *Handbook of Bereavement: Theory, Research and Intervention.* Cambridge: Cambridge University Press.
9 Sanders, C.M. (1988) Risk factors in bereavement outcome. *Journal of Social Issues,* 44: 97–111.
10 Parkes, C.M. (1990) Risk factors in bereavement: implications for the prevention and treatment of pathologic grief. *Psychiatric Annals,* 20: 308–13.
11 Parkes, C.M. (1990) Bereavement counselling: does it work? *British Medical Journal,* 281: 3–6.
12 Parkes, C.M. (1993) Bereavement, in D. Doyle, G.W.C. Hanks and N. Macdonald (eds) *Oxford Textbook of Palliative Medicine.* Oxford: Oxford University Press, 1993.

13 Lattanzi-Licht, M.E. (1989) Bereavement services: practice and problems. *The Hospice Journal*, 5: 1–28.
14 Parkes, C.M. (1981) Op. cit.
15 Lattanzi-Licht, M.E. (1989) Op. cit.
16 Gibson, D.W. and Graham, D. (1991) *Bereavement risk assessment in Australian hospice care centres: a survey.* Dissertation, Ballarat University College, Australia.
17 Wilkes, E. (1993) Op. cit.
18 *Directory of Hospice Services in the UK and Ireland 1992* (1992). Sydenham: St Christopher's Hospice Information Service.
19 Gibson, D.W. and Graham, D. (1991) Op. cit.
20 Parkes, C.M. (1993) Op. cit.
21 Littlewood, J. (1992) *Aspects of Grief.* London: Routledge.
22 Gibson, D.W. and Graham, D. (1991) Op. cit.
23 Lattanzi-Licht, M.E. (1989) Op. cit.
24 Ibid.
25 Parkes, C.M. (1981) Op. cit.
26 Beckwick, B.E., Beckwith, S.K., Gray, T.L. *et al.* (1990) Identification of spouses at high risk during bereavement: a preliminary assessment of Parkes and Weiss's Risk Index. *Hospice Journal*, 6: 35–45.
27 Levy, L.H., Derby, J.F. and Martinowski, K.S. (1992) The question of who participates in bereavement research and the bereavement risk index. *Omega*, 25: 225–38.
28 Ibid.
29 *Sir Michael Sobell House Demographic Data 1988–1991.* Oxford: Sobell Publications. (1992).
30 Wilkes, E. (1993) Op. cit.
31 Ibid.

Acknowledgements

We would like to thank everyone who responded to the survey and Angela Holly for assistance in coding the data.

Reprinted from Payne, S.A. and Relf, M. (1994) The assessment of need for bereavement follow-up in palliative and hospice care. *Palliative Medicine*, 12: 197–203.

Clinical audit and organizational audit in palliative care

IRENE J. HIGGINSON

Introduction

Critical appraisal of palliative medicine began in the late 1970s and early 1980s, perhaps because it was one of the newest specialities in cancer care and thus had much to prove. The very first modern hospices evaluated care, compared care between hospices or home care teams and assessed many aspects of care, particularly the control of pain and other symptoms.[1-8] Such evaluations were necessary to justify the continuation of the hospice and to demonstrate effective methods to control symptoms.[9]

Although evaluation showed the value of a few 'pioneer' hospices and teams or of symptom control methods, these benefits cannot be assumed for all units. Palliative medicine has expanded rapidly during the past 20 years. Expansion has brought with it great variations in practice[10-12] and often very little or no information on the value of some practices. Audit is needed to ensure that care is optimal in many units, old and new.

Effective audit is a cyclical activity, with three principal stages. The first is to set standards for the delivery of care. The second is to observe practice and compare it with the standards. This often demonstrates successes, but it also shows failings and need for change. The third stage feeds the results back to those providing care, so that new or modified standards can be set. The audit cycle is then repeated anew.[13-17] The cycle can be entered at any point; for example, it is possible to begin by observing practice and acting on the results and then proceed to setting standards.

This chapter has been slightly revised by Professor Higginson for this publication.

Table 16.1 Definitions of medical, clinical and nursing audit

Type of audit	Definition
Medical	Systematic critical analysis of the quality of medical care including the procedures used for diagnosis and treatment, the use of resources and the resulting outcome and quality of life of the patient[18]
Clinical	Systematic critical analysis of the quality of clinical care including the procedures used for diagnosis and treatment, the use of resources and the resulting outcome and quality of life of the patient. Clinical audit is like medical audit but involves all professionals and volunteers rather than only doctors
Nursing	Methods by nurses compare their actual practice against agreed guidelines and identify areas for improving their care
Organizational	Development of organizational standards and examining a unit's (e.g. hospital, hospice) progress towards meeting those standards

Clinical audit

Clinical audit has grown out of separate medical and nursing audits. It is most suited to areas of care where doctors, nurses and other staff work in teams, sharing decision making (see Table 16.1 for definitions). In palliative care, where ideally the patients' concerns are discussed by all staff, clinical, rather than medical, audit is most appropriate.[19]

Clinical audit can assess the structure (the resources, e.g. staffing numbers and qualifications), the process (the use of resources, such as number of visits, drugs prescribed), the output (e.g. throughput, discharge rate) or outcome (the change in quality of life or health status as a result of care, such as pain control).[20]

Although palliative care cannot be audited with the usual measures of mortality and morbidity, an array of measures is now available (Table 16.2). These cover both simple aspects of process, such as documentation standards and procedures followed, and more complicated aspects of outcome, such as symptom control, coordination, communication and psychosocial problems.

The audits are at very different stages of use and development. Three – the Support Team Assessment Schedule (STAS), the Trent Documentation Standards and the Regional Study of Care of the Dying – have been used in a wide variety of settings or in different regions of the UK. Items in the STAS have also been tested for validity and reliability, the Edmonton Symptom Assessment Scale[21] has been subject to similar testing against STAS. For other measures, modifications are being made. Guidelines for good practice and audit measures from the Royal College of Physicians,[22] although developed many years ago, have not yet been used.[23]

This range of available measures and methods for audit in palliative care should provide most clinicians with a choice for their own practice. The setting of standards and the development of instruments can be a lengthy process, and it is probably better to adapt measures that are available or being tested, if possible.

Organizational audit

Organizational audit can be seen as the developmental and voluntary stage towards accreditation. In the UK, the King's Fund Centre (1990) developed a project initially called 'Accreditation UK' and later called 'Organizational Audit', which worked voluntarily with National Health Service and private hospitals to agree to a lengthy document of standards. Organizational standards were developed because of evidence of organizational variation, which limits the quality of care. These include administrative delays and uncoordinated care.[24,25] Organizational standards need to be simple enough to be monitored by an external inspector if they are to be eventually used for accreditation. Organizational audit and accreditation are usually developed in three stages:[26]

1 developing organizational standards of the systems and process of care;
2 implementation of the standards by the hospices, hospitals or units included;
3 evaluation of compliance with the standards, usually by external inspectors.

The first stage in the development of standards can often be quite lengthy, because the standards need to be agreed on and written in clear, non-ambiguous language and then tested to determine if the standards can distinguish between good and suboptimal practice. If the standards can detect only the poorest practice, then they may lower standards to just above this level, because units will not need to strive higher.

The Cancer Relief Macmillan Fund developed organizational audit for palliative care, following the same type of development as the King's Fund project. A small working group consisting of six regional coordinators for palliative care, five of whom were nurses, and a representative from Cancer Relief Macmillan Fund, developed an initial draft of standards. These were modified and piloted in several hospices in the UK. The 11 standards and their purposes are:[27]

- service values – a statement of service values and objectives related to the palliative care service guides the organization and delivery of high-quality care;
- organization and management – the palliative care service or organization is managed efficiently to ensure patients and families receive suitable and effective multidisciplinary care;
- organizational and operational policy – organizational and operational policies reflect current knowledge and principles and are consistent with the requirements of statutory bodies, purchasing authorities and service objectives;
- physical environment for care – the physical environment is safe and accommodates individual and shared needs;
- self-determination and climate for care – the caring environment for patients and families is conducive to independence, self-esteem and participation in daily life;
- direct patient and family care – professional staff ensure that patient and family needs are assessed, planned, implemented and evaluated on an individual basis;
- multidisciplinary working and team work – a range of skills is available to meet service goals, and specific contributions are identified and integrated, from both within and outside the service;
- staffing and skill mix – good employment practices are in place, and staffing levels are systematically determined in order to meet service needs;
- education, training and staff development – staff are developed and have access to programmes of education and training that reflect the different levels of activity and practice necessary to meet service goals, provide appropriate care and respond to change;
- staff support – the possible emotional effects on staff involved in palliative care are recognized, and there are resources for the provision of appropriate support;
- ethics and law – there is guidance and support for staff to comply with statutory requirements and use a systematic approach to decision making where ethical and legal status issues are involved.

Each of these 11 standards has a series of questions that are used by a team of external inspectors to determine the extent to which each standard is achieved. The validity, reliability, practicality and sensitivity of the questions are unreported.

Potential uses of clinical and organizational audit

Clinical and organizational audits are used in different ways and have different benefits and drawbacks. Clinical audit is normally developed by the

Figure 16.1 Proposed benefits of internal and external audit showing aspects where internal audit has most benefits

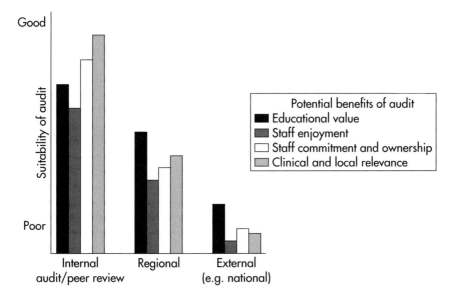

clinical staff working with patients and families in one or a few units and tends to be locally based and relevant. However, national clinical audits are possible, as for example the study of care of the dying (although this is more costly than local audits because it uses external interviewers), or the Palliative Care Core Standards (Table 16.2).[28] By contrast, organizational audit is usually developed by a national or regional body, with the long-term goal of being used to compare units or for the accreditation of units. Thus, whereas clinical audit is usually locally owned and controlled, organizational audit is usually externally inspected and controlled.

The relative benefits of local internal audits versus external national audits are estimated in Figs. 16.1 and 16.2. Local clinical audit brings with it a high educational value[29] because of the involvement and commitment of staff, and is probably more enjoyable for staff taking part. It can also be made relevant to local problems and population, such as the needs of different ethnic groups. However, it does not lend itself easily to national standards or external inspections. How could an external inspector review clinical outcomes, such as pain control, without using independent interviews of patients or families in care, which would be extremely costly? External inspectors, however, can fairly easily review the organizational aspects of care, such as policies and staff training. They can be more confident in their comparison of the units' organizational standards and provide guidelines for setting contracts between purchasers of care and providers.

Figure 16.2   Proposed benefits of internal and external audit showing aspects where external audit has most benefits

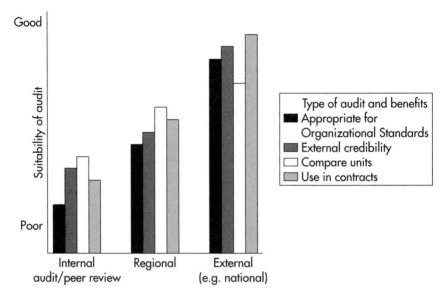

How much audit is cost-effective?

Given the differing potential uses of clinical and organizational audit, it could be argued that both should be employed. The next question is, How much of each is appropriate? The most important constraint is cost. Both clinical and organizational audits have cost implications in terms of the time for staff to take part in the audit, the time to collect and analyse the audit data, discuss results and agree on the change in action.[30] This takes time away from direct patient care and, although it may be of benefit to patients and families in the long term, short-term difficulties may occur. Sufficient time needs to be allocated for staff to be involved in audit. In practice, only one or a few audits can take place at any one time.

To achieve value for money from audit, audit needs to be cost-effective, just as much as clinical care needs to be cost-effective. The audit must result in improved outcomes of care for patients and their families. The extent to which different audits have achieved this is now considered to suggest the next steps for audit.

Next steps for organizational audit

In theory, organizational audit is valuable if its framework indicates the systems and processes necessary to ensure an efficient and effective service

Table 16.2 Some clinical audits for palliative care

Name and source	Number of items and aspects of care included	How developed and setting	Stage of development
Palliative care: guidelines for good practice and audit measures (Royal College of Physicians 1991)[31]	29 items covering: admission policy (5) clinical management (6) support of patient and family (5) communication (4) documentation and administration (9) *Structure and process of care*	Working group of the Royal College of Physicians, which met to consider key papers and then corresponded In-patient hospices	Items are listed but not tested in practice
The Support Team Assessment Schedule (Higginson 1993)[32]	17 items covering: pain and symptoms (2) patient anxiety, insight and spiritual (3) family anxiety and insight (2) planning affairs (2) communication (3) home services (3) support of other professionals (2) *Outcomes and intermediate outcomes*	Collaboration with five support teams and revised in light of presentations at professional meetings, observation of palliative care, interviews with patients and families Now used in different settings	Used widely; time to complete on one patient averages two minutes; validated to ensure professional ratings reflect patient views; reliable. Testing use of individual items, expanding symptom assessment and database under way
Palliative Care Core Standards (Trent Hospice Audit Group 1992)[33]	6 standard statements and 56 process and outcome items: collaboration with other agencies (8) symptom control (6) patient/carer information (9) emotional support (11) bereavement care and support (13) specialist education/training for staff (9) *Structure, process and outcomes*	Regional collaboration of hospice and home care units In-patient hospice and community	Standards and measures developed and are being revised following a pilot study to evaluate and review the core standards and to determine the criteria for the standards usage

Table 16.2 (cont'd)

Name and source	Number of items and aspects of care included	How developed and setting	Stage of development
Care of people with a terminal illness (National Association of Health Authorities and Trusts 1991)[34]	10 standards for contracts covering policies, provision, consumer participation, education, direct care, attitude, skills and mix of staff. 10 areas with numbers of standards for care in nursing homes *Structure and process*	Advisory group	Standards are published but measures of the standards are not listed
Documentation standards (Catterall 1993)[35]	62 documentation standards covering: general (4) referral details (23) admission assessment and progress (26) after death (5) after discharge (4) *Process*	Six medical directors In-patient hospice	Standards went through three rounds of testing, improvement and revision Have been used to audit care in six units

Study	Description	Setting	Status
Regional study of care of the dying (Addington-Hall and McCarthy 1993)[36]	Questionnaire administered by the person who knew most about the patients, approximately seven months after their deaths; it assesses services received, symptoms during the last year of life, communication, satisfaction with care and mental status of the carer *Process and outcomes*	Adapted from studies by Cartwright et al. (1973)[37] and Cartwright and Seale (1990)[38]	It builds on information collected 30 years ago and fifteen years ago so that patterns of care and symptoms can be compared The new study has interviewed the carers of 3500 people who died in 20 districts in England
Edmonton Symptom Assessment System (Bruera et al. 1991)[39]	9 visual analogue scales: pain, activity, nausea, depression, anxiety, drowsiness, appetite, well-being, shortness of breath *Outcome*	By members of hospice service In-patient hospice	In use and being validated
Finlay (1993)[40]	Topic audits including: blood transfusion drug chart recording, restlessness, pressure sores, communication *Process and outcome*	By members of hospice service In-patient hospice	Several completed cycles, but audit only used locally Standardized clinical records developed

to patients and their families or carers and a good working environment for staff. However, an ideal structure does not necessarily result in an ideal process and thereby an ideal outcome of care for the patient. Unfortunately, the ideal structure is not proven by research methods: studies to compare structure of care do not exist, nor are any planned.

The formation of standards therefore depends on the views of experts and on commonly accepted good practice, such as general beliefs that multidisciplinary working, education and training programmes and staff support systems facilitate 'good' care. Although it can be argued that without these systems, 'good' care may be difficult or impossible to provide, it is not proven that the presence of these systems alone results in improved care. How much education (and what type, by what level of skilled educators, on what types of staff with what system of beliefs and background) needs to be determined before we can be sure exactly what education is needed. This limits the value of organizational audit and suggests that large resources should not be dedicated to providing minute details of the structure of care, which itself has an unknown value.

Furthermore, if experts, rather than scientific evidence, are to decide which procedures are to be advocated in organizational audit, then who is an 'expert'? What are their experiences, backgrounds and qualifications? Where should they work? In palliative care, it must be argued that a multiprofessional panel would be needed to agree on standards. The composition of the Cancer Relief Macmillan Fund working party can be criticized for including an insufficiently broad range of professionals beyond nurses. Although other professionals were included in the consultation stage, to what degree their opinions carried weight is not known.

Setting the pace for the organizational audit of palliative care in the future will require research into the different outcomes produced by different structures of care. If the audit is to develop into a system of national accreditation, proof of the patient benefits from the organizational audit, by completing a cycle, and the costs and practicalities will also be needed.

Next steps for clinical audit

There is a longer history for clinical audit than for organizational audit, and more is known about its strengths and failures. One of the most fruitful approaches appears to be to combine process and outcome information in the audit. This will allow staff to determine both the result of care and what process caused that result. This approach can give clear information on what aspects of care need to be changed. Finlay[41] audited the use of blood transfusion in terminal cancer and combined audit data on the indications and clinical practice for blood transfusion (process) with information on the patient's symptoms.

The results of clinical audit, which provide process and outcome data, can be used to develop clinical algorithms to predict symptoms or to develop treatment protocols. To develop prognostic indicators to predict which patients were likely to suffer uncontrollable pain, Bruera et al.[42] developed the Edmonton staging system for cancer pain. Using this algorithm, earlier treatment can be planned, and patients at risk of uncontrolled pain can be referred early to specialist treatment centres. Clinical audit demonstrated that dyspnoea (breathlessness) remained uncontrolled during palliative care in the majority of cases.[43] Primary or secondary cancer in the lung or pleura and existing dyspnoea predicted over 50 per cent of the cases in which severe unrelieved dyspnoea developed. However, using information from the audit assessment in our community support team, we developed a clinical algorithm with higher sensitivity and specificity.[44] Piloting the audit in a new group of patients correctly classified 94 per cent into those likely, or not, to develop uncontrolled dyspnoea. We are now testing the robustness of this algorithm in a larger group of patients, using data from several services. Next steps for clinical audit, apart from ensuring completion of the audit cycle, would surely be for clinicians to develop algorithms that assist in the planning and management of patient care.

One of the main dangers of local clinical audits is duplication of work, particularly the setting of standards. Each service feels a need to set its own standards, so that these are locally relevant. However, as demonstrated above, standard setting takes considerable time. There is now a need to bring together the results and methods used in local clinical audits and to compare findings. This could occur within regions or nationally. In this way, clinicians can learn from each other's results, test each other's methods and avoid duplication.

Management and evaluation of audit

Shaw[45] outlined ten requirements for the successful management of audit: intention, leadership, participation, control, method, resources, guidelines, comparison, conclusions and feedback. Anecdotal reports of audit failure have often been attributed to poor management of the introduction and continuation of audit. Hunt[46] reported difficulties when staff perceived that the audit was imposed upon them, and they were not given sufficient opportunity to discuss the findings. McKee[47] reported the value of 'selling' audit to staff and allowing ample time for discussion and agreement of methods.

At first, it may seem unnecessary to assess whether audit actually benefits patient care. However, to ensure audit is cost-effective, it must prove to be useful. Audit itself is far too rarely appraised. Few systematic assessments of the benefits of audit, whether it led to changes in practice or staff's appraisals of the audit, have been published. Hayes[48] reported an anonymous questionnaire survey of staff after one year of audit. Three quarters of the staff wanted to continue with the audit more or less as it was, but criticisms included that the measure used did not give a full picture of the patient and that the results of audit were not reported quickly enough. Hayes concluded that a very simple first evaluation should be carried out after three months and repeated at regular intervals. Although many units do claim to discuss the audits informally and appraise these, Hayes demonstrated that a more formal and systematic anonymous evaluation identified some problems hitherto unrecognized. Evaluation of audit must surely be seen as an integral part of its introduction and management.

Conclusions

Audit approaches and methods are now well advanced in palliative care, especially in clinical audit. Clinicians are presented with a choice of possibilities, rather than having to undertake much of the development themselves. Practical approaches include the Support Team Assessment Schedule and the Edmonton Symptom Assessment Scale (both of which either have been validated or are being tested for this) and Finlay's topic audits. Clinical audits that take place after death are probably more costly, but are still possible, and again measures are available. Apart from completing the audit cycle, clinical audit can look to developing clinical protocols for treatment or algorithms to predict patient problems and the need for specialized care. Organizational audit is less well advanced, and we need research to determine what patient benefit results from the advocated structures of care. An unanswered question remains, Who should be the 'experts' who decide what constitutes an ideal structure? Various organizational audit and accreditation systems are now being tested in the UK. The results are likely to provide some very useful data to assist this debate. The areas of management and evaluation of audit are perhaps least explored but appear to be vital for cost-effective audit.

The World Health Organization[49] recommended that palliative care needs to extend to include cancer patients earlier in care, rather than those just near to death. If this occurs, then palliative care audit should also include patients at an earlier stage of their illness, and the audit itself could be used as a means for clinical dialogue and comparison of care. Palliative medicine could take the lead in encouraging this, promoting methods among medical and surgical colleagues.

References

1 Parkes, C.M. (1978) Home or hospital? Terminal care as seen by surviving spouses. *Journal of the Royal College of General Practitioners*, 28: 19–30.

2 Parkes, C.M. (1979a) Terminal care: evaluation of in-patient service at St Christopher's Hospice. Part I: Views of surviving spouse on effects of the service on the patient. *Postgraduate Medical Journal*, 55: 517–22.

3 Parkes, C.M. (1979b) Terminal care: evaluation of in-patient service at St Christopher's Hospice. Part II: Self-assessments of effects of the service on surviving spouses. *Postgraduate Medical Journal*, 55: 523–7.

4 Parkes, C.M. (1980) Terminal care: evaluation of an advisory domiciliary service at St Christopher's Hospice. *Postgraduate Medical Journal*, 56: 685–9.

5 Hinton, J. (1979) A comparison of places and policies for terminal care. *Lancet*, i: 29–32.

6 Kane, R., Wales, J., Bernstein, L., Leibowitz, A. and Kaplan, S. (1984) A randomised controlled trial of hospice care. *Lancet*, i: 890–4.

7 Kane, R., Klein, S., Bernstein, L., Rothenberg, R. and Wales, J. (1985) Hospice role in alleviating the emotional stress of terminal patients and their families. *Medical Care*, 23: 189–97.

8 Ward, A.W.M. (1985) *Home Care Services for the Terminally Ill.* Sheffield: Medical Care Research Unit, Department of Community Medicine, University of Sheffield Medical School.

9 Higginson, I. and McCarthy, M. (1989a) Evaluation of palliative care: steps to quality assurance? *Palliative Medicine*, 3: 267–74.

10 Ward, A.W.M. (1987) Home care services – an alternative to hospices? *Community Medicine*, 9: 47–54.

11 Kirkham, S. (1992) Bed occupancy, patient throughput and size of independent hospice units in the UK. *Palliative Medicine*, 6: 47–53.

12 Higginson, I. (1993) Palliative care: a review of past challenges and future trends. *Journal of Public Health*, 15: 3–8.

13 Shaw, C.D. (1980) Aspect of audit, 1: The background. *British Medical Journal*, 280: 1256–8.

14 Shaw, C. (1989) *Medical Audit – A Hospital Handbook.* London: King's Fund Centre.

15 Department of Health (1989) *Working for Patients: Medical Audit*, working paper 6. London: Her Majesty's Stationery Office.

16 Department of Health (1990) *Medical Audit in the Hospital and Community Health Services*, draft health circular. London: Department of Health.

17 Department of Health (1991) *Medical Audit in the Hospital and Community Health Services.* London: Her Majesty's Stationery Office.

18 Department of Health (1989) Op. cit.

19 Ford, G. (1990) Constructive audit. *Palliative Medicine*, 4: 1–2.

20 Donabedian, A. (1980) *Explorations in Quality Assessment and Monitoring, Volume 1. The Definition of Quality and Approaches to its Assessment.* Michigan, MI: Health Administration Press.

21 Bruera, E. and MacDonald, S. (1993) Audit methods: the Edmonton Symptom Assessment System, in I. Higginson (ed.) *Clinical Audit in Palliative Care.* Oxford: Radcliffe Medical Press.

22 Royal College of Physicians (1991) *Palliative Care – Guidelines for Good Practice and Audit Measures*. London: Royal College of Physicians.

23 Hopkins, A., personal communication.

24 King's Fund Centre (1990) *Organisational Audit (Accreditation UK): Standards for an Acute Hospital*. London: King's Fund Centre.

25 Shaw, C. (1992) *Speciality Medical Audit*. London: King's Fund Centre.

26 King's Fund Centre (1990) Op. cit.

27 Cancer Relief Macmillan Fund (1992) Organisational audit for palliative care services. A working document. London: Cancer Relief Macmillan Fund.

28 Trent Hospice Audit Group (1992) *Palliative Care Core Standards: A Multidisciplinary Approach*, c/o Nightingale Macmillan Continuing Care Unit, Trinity Street, Derby.

29 Coles, C. (1990) Making audit truly educational. *Postgraduate Medical Journal*, 66 (Supplement): S32–S36.

30 Shaw, C. (1992) Op. cit.

31 Royal College of Physicians (1991) Op. cit.

32 Higginson, I. (1993) Op. cit.

33 Trent Hospice Audit Group (1992) Op. cit.

34 National Association of Health Authorities and Trusts (1991) *Care of People with a Terminal Illness*. Birmingham: National Association of Health Authorities and Trusts.

35 Catterall, R.A. (1993) Audit methods: regional documentation standards, in I. Higginson (ed.) *Clinical Audit in Palliative Care*. Oxford: Radcliffe Medical Press.

36 Addington-Hall, J. and McCarthy, M. (1993) Audit methods: views of the family after the death, in I. Higginson (ed.) *Clinical Audit in Palliative Care*. Oxford: Radcliffe Medical Press.

37 Cartwright, A., Hockey, L. and Anderson, J.L. (1973) *Life Before Death*. London: Routledge and Kegan Paul.

38 Cartwright, A. and Seale, C. (1990) *The Natural History of a Survey: An Account of the Methodological Issues Encountered in a Study of Life Before Death*. London: King Edward's Hospital Fund.

39 Bruera, E., Kuehn, N., Miller, M., Selmser, P. and MacMillan, K. (1991) The Edmonton symptom assessment system (ESAS): a simple method for the assessment of palliative care patients. *Journal of Palliative Care*, 7: 6–9.

40 Finlay, I. (1993) Audit experience: views of a hospice director, in I. Higginson (ed.) *Clinical Audit in Palliative Care*. Oxford: Radcliffe Medical Press.

41 Ibid.

42 Bruera, E., MacMillan, K., Hanson, J. and MacDonald, R. (1989) The Edmonton staging system for cancer pain: preliminary report. *Pain*, 37: 203–9.

43 Higginson, I. and McCarthy, M. (1989b) Measuring symptoms in terminal cancer: are pain and dyspnoea controlled? *Journal of the Royal Society of Medicine*, 82: 264–7.

44 Wade, A., Higginson, I. and McCarthy, M. (1988) The use of self audit to predict dyspnoea in terminally ill cancer patients. *Social Science and Medicine*, 56 [Abstract].

45 Shaw, C. (1989) Op. cit.

46 Hunt, I. (1993) Audit methods: palliative care core standards, in I. Higginson (ed.) *Clinical Audit in Palliative Care*. Oxford: Radcliffe Medical Press.

47 McKee, E. (1993) Audit experience: a nurse manager in home care, in I. Higginson (ed.) *Clinical Audit in Palliative Care*. Oxford: Radcliffe Medical Press.

48 Hayes, A. (1993) Audit experience: assessing staff's views, in I. Higginson (ed.) *Clinical Audit in Palliative Care*. Oxford: Radcliffe Medical Press.

49 World Health Organization Expert Committee (1990) *Cancer Pain Relief and Palliative Care*, World Health Organization Technical Report Series 804. Geneva: WHO.

Acknowledgement

Higginson, I. (1994) Palliative medicine: problem areas in pain and symptom management. *Cancer Surveys*, 21: 233–45.

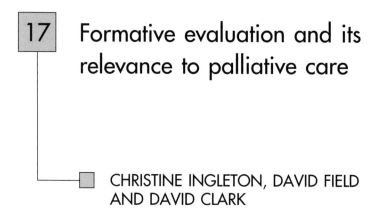

17 Formative evaluation and its relevance to palliative care

CHRISTINE INGLETON, DAVID FIELD
AND DAVID CLARK

Introduction

For the most part, the evaluation of health care and attempts to improve the quality of health care have drawn upon quantitative methods of research. However, for many questions, and in many health care specialities, quantitative methods of evaluation may be neither practical, desirable, nor ethical. Qualitative methods may be more appropriate when evaluators are attempting to 'open up' a new field of study[1] or are concerned to illuminate and understand issues in an ever-changing context. Various qualitative methods have been developed which potentially hold out a number of possibilities within the area of palliative care.[2] Qualitative case study evaluation is one such example. In this chapter, key characteristics of this methodological approach are presented and explained, and illustrated by reference to the evaluation of two palliative care services. More specifically, the chapter will focus upon the *process* of conducting this type of evaluation in the context of palliative care. For this reason the evaluation findings are presented elsewhere.[3–6]

Methodological approaches to evaluation

The literature concerned with evaluation reveals two distinct methodological approaches, namely summative and formative evaluation. That distinction is primarily one of purpose. Summative evaluation seeks to draw causal inferences about the effects of a programme or intervention. Evaluators working in this way will seek to remain detached from the politics and activities they study, in order to identify clear and immeasurable outcomes of the services being provided. They will often do this by adopting an approach which relies upon the methodology of the controlled trial, for example by comparing the outcomes and outputs from control and experimental groups. In practice, however, there are problems, especially in the evaluation of health care. For example, it is difficult (and may be impossible) to locate any clear statement of the service aims, particularly in the context of a newly operational service. Frequently, the overall shape and function of a service changes rapidly over time, particularly if it is an innovative service. Also there may be differing views from various interest groups about what constitutes a 'good' or a 'bad' service; each group may have a legitimate, but disparate interpretation of events.[7,8] Taken together, these circumstances preclude experimental approaches to evaluation, and so evaluators have looked to other methods as a way of overcoming these problems.

Formative evaluation offers one such approach. Formative evaluation pays more attention to the social context, and the social and political processes which are associated with the implementation of a particular service, and looks at the relationship between service objectives and their outcomes. It is sensitive to unintended, as well as intended outcomes. Working in this mode, evaluators do not 'distance' themselves from those being 'evaluated' but involve themselves actively at key stages of design, data collection and analysis. Evaluators are also part of the process and acknowledge themselves as such, hence they use the term 'reflexive' to describe their role in shaping and interpreting events. Formative evaluation has as its main thrust the provision of information, which seeks to improve the delivery of the service and typically uses an eclectic approach to gather data.[9–12] Although it relies to a large extent on qualitative methods, quantitative methods such as closed format questionnaires may also be used. Formative evaluation has become synonymous with the practice of qualitative evaluation. The bases of formative evaluation are:

- the use of case studies;
- the use of multiple methods of data collection;
- the acknowledgement of the role/influence of evaluators in the evaluation process (reflexivity);
- an evaluation as a political process;
- the emphasis placed on utility.

The use of case studies

Qualitative evaluations may often take the form of in-depth case studies. Case studies provide the method of choice when the phenomenon under study is not readily distinguishable from its context; they are particularly useful when studying a unique situation in a changing context.[13–14] The two services we studied in this way were King's Mill Hospice and Beaumond House, and both possessed all these characteristics. Both developed their strategic and operational plans for service development against a background of continuing policy and legislative change at national, regional and district level. Both had novel features in the provision of their services. In the case of King's Mill, the hospice has an unusual (possibly unique) organizational structure, bringing together the work of a National Health Service trust and a charitable trust in partnership. Beaumond House had adopted a model based on the principles of community care ideas, which were somewhat novel and not within the mainstream of hospice care. Both organizations were themselves part of complex systems of care for terminally ill patients and their carers. Therefore, the perceptions of groups 'outside' the organizations, such as the primary health care teams, had an important bearing upon its operation and any planned evaluation.

King's Mill Hospice, based in Sutton-in-Ashfield, near Mansfield, provides in-patient beds, day care places, home sitting and loan of specialist equipment, and a range of therapies including physiotherapy, occupational therapy, complementary therapies and counselling. The hospice is located in a purpose-built unit at the edge of a general hospital site. Beaumond House is situated 30 km from King's Mill Hospice, in the market town of Newark. It provides a community-based model of care with day places, respite beds, bereavement care, and education and information for the local community. In common with many other palliative care services then, both organizations offered such a variety of services and involved so many different professional groups, as well as volunteers, patients and carers, that no single criterion of evaluation would suffice. Additionally, as in all evaluation studies, there were multiple, frequently competing perspectives and potential audiences, comprising groups who had a vested interest in the service being evaluated (the 'stakeholders').

The use of multiple methods

An important feature of the case study is the use of multiple methods and sources of evidence to ensure rigour. This frequently takes the form of triangulation.[15–18] These are illustrated in Table 17.1.

In both studies, we made use of different methods of triangulation. Triangulation has its roots in navigational, military or surveying contexts,[19] where it refers to the use of two known and fixed points in order to locate the position of a third. In the context of research, this approach dates back to Campbell and Fiske[20] who argued the need to measure a single concept in a number of different ways. This early application lodged triangulation

Table 17.1   Methods of triangulation

Type	Meaning
Theoretical triangulation	Involves the use of several different 'frames of reference' or perspectives in the analysis
Data triangulation	Involves the use of different data sources for the same phenomenon
Method triangulation	Involves employing different methods in order to address the same phenomenon
Analysis triangulation	The same data set is analysed using two or more different techniques
Investigator or interdisciplinary triangulation	Perspectives from a range of disciplines are brought to bear on the topic of inquiry

within the positivist paradigm of measurement,[21] although in recent times it has become the cornerstone of qualitative inquiry. Triangulation offers flexibility and an in-depth approach that is not always possible with simple one-method designs. But, there may be difficulties in replicating studies and an increased danger of lack of focus. To achieve methodological and data triangulation, we used a wide range of qualitative and quantitative methods from a range of different data sources (Figure 17.1).

The aim of the two studies was to describe and understand the day-to-day work of the hospice and the quality of its services, through an analysis of how it related to other services in its locality, matters of strategic planning and the views of those who supported its work in the wider community. In other words, the aim was to achieve a dynamic and 'holistic' view of the hospice in its wider social context. Thus, we started with broad questions and aims rather than by posing precise questions at the outset. These questions were then refined and became more specific in the course of field work and the parallel process of data analysis.

We carried out interviews, survey work and non-participant observation, and inspected written documents such as minutes of meetings, correspondence, business plans and organizational charts. A systematic approach to data gathering was adopted. For example, if we were confronted with conflicting accounts between different stakeholders in survey responses, these were probed in in-depth interviews to obtain possible explanations. Another way of checking the credibility of our interpretations was through the use of respondent validation. That is, the analysis of the settings that emerged was presented to stakeholders for their reaction. Using this technique, our analysis was refined and improved by stakeholder feedback. It is important

Figure 17.1 Newark and District hospice aid: convergence and multiple methods and sources

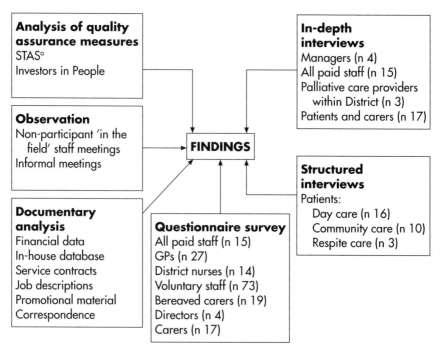

a Higginson, I., Wade, A. and McCarthy, M. (1992) Effectiveness of two palliative care support teams, *The Journal of Public Health Medicine*, 1: 50–6.

to note that the perspectives of the various groups are not dealt with evenly within each of the two case studies (for example, Figure 17.1). This was because of the varying emphasis placed by certain groups according to their perceived significance to the service. There were two main reasons for this variation. The first stemmed from the underlying philosophy of evaluation which underlines the importance of stakeholders focusing on what they considered to be substantive issues. Time and resources, as well as methodological considerations, were also an issue when focusing methods and sampling options into a framework which was manageable, practical and credible. For example, the length of the project at Beaumond House was six months, compared to four months at King's Mill. Thus, a more consistent period of time was spent in an observational capacity at Beaumond House which, it could be argued, provided a 'thicker description' of context[22] than was possible at King's Mill. Conversely, the perspective of voluntary staff at King's Mill was canvassed using a wider variety of methods and was subject to a more in-depth analysis than that of the voluntary staff at Beaumond House. At King's Mill, the role of voluntary staff was thought to merit particular attention by the commissioners as, compared with other hospice organizations, King's Mill makes greater use of such staff than is usual.[23] Also, an unusual aspect of voluntary staff at King's Mill is that day-to-day management of voluntary staff teams is undertaken by the voluntary staff themselves.

Thus, our exploratory and interpretative framework was not imposed on the data, but derived from it in an iterative process over the course of the evaluation.

Interprofessional triangulation was accomplished by involving a small team of evaluators, each with a special interest in specific issues and with particular methodological skills. The two multiprofessional teams were comprised of individuals from the disciplines of medicine, nursing, sociology and psychology. We found that the multiprofessional orientation of the teams, reflecting the multiprofessional perspective of palliative care, was essential to the credibility of the findings. The challenge in the future, however, may be a shift from multiprofessional to interprofessional working. Multiprofessional evaluation, like multiprofessional care, is based on the premise that each member of the team has a different training and, therefore, brings different skills to bear.[24] Here coordination is the key. Interprofessional evaluation, while not repudiating the importance of specific skills and characteristics, seeks to blur academic and professional boundaries. Thus a willingness to share responsibility becomes the focus.[25] Much is spoken of the concept of interprofessional research, especially in palliative care circles. The literature on collaborative research, though sparse in both volume and critique, reveals that there are various ways in which collaboration can be configured. For example, collaboration can occur between clinicians and academics,[26] between various organizations[27] and between various professional groups. At King's Mill, for example, there was a matrix of collaboration between clinicians and academics, three different professional groups, a hospice and two university departments and finally (and unusually) between the evaluation team and key stakeholders.

In using any method of triangulation, the evaluator is often faced with findings which may reveal a divergence of opinion among stakeholders. As a consequence, results may point toward different conclusions. This need not necessarily be a problem, and it can convey benefits. For example, in some circumstances, widely differing opinions are themselves important and these were considered in our evaluation reports.[28]

Evaluator reflexivity

Underpinning formative evaluation is an acceptance that evaluators are part of the social world they are examining. Rather than engaging in attempts to eliminate the effect of the evaluator, 'reflexive evaluators' accept that they are an integral factor in the data collection, analysis and findings. This should not necessarily be considered a source of bias, but does indicate the need for self-awareness. Because the observer is part of the social world in which the study takes place, the evaluator thus becomes an active participant within the narrative. We would argue that reflexive observation allows a greater depth of material to be studied *in context*, than if the observer is 'distanced' from the participants and the field of inquiry. In contrast, evaluators working within a positivist framework would seek to 'control' or minimize the so-called 'halo' or 'Hawthorne effect'.[29]

The process of reflexivity is not merely something located in the design stage of a study or evaluation, but continues throughout all phases of the process from planning the evaluation to the dissemination of findings.[30] For this reason, it is appropriate for the evaluators to examine their own premises and to make them explicit in the report. Completion of a reflexive journal or diary, in which the evaluators on a daily basis, or as needed, record a variety of information about their role in constructing the data, provides a way of recording events throughout the process and of monitoring the performance of evaluators. In our studies, the reflexive account in the evaluation report was offered as evidence of validity of what is reported.

Evaluation as a political process

Politics and evaluation are inextricably linked. To begin with, an evaluation is generally commissioned by the agency responsible for the service, not the recipients of its efforts. In the case of King's Mill Hospice, the evaluation was commissioned by the agency responsible for the service, not the recipients of the service. By contrast, at Beaumond House, the evaluation was commissioned and funded by the purchaser. This has important ramifications for all stages of the evaluation, as several parties have a 'stake' in the content and form of the report. If evaluations are seen as having a role in 'improving services' then it follows that evaluators must be concerned with the political aspects of the evaluation. In the health care context, stakeholders range from purchasers to providers, in what may be a climate of competition, to intended 'users' of the service such as patients and relatives. Establishing where 'ownership' of the evaluation lies requires clarification at the outset of the study as this may not always be apparent, as we found in our study at King's Mill Hospice. For this reason, different approaches to negotiation of evaluation protocols, aims, access, evaluators' roles and modes of dissemination become necessary. This of course may prove no easy task. It is important that, in the initial discussions and contract proposal, the degree of control that the commissioners and funders subsequently have over content and publication is clarified. Some commissioning agents or commissioning bodies may expect a power of veto, and modification or

exclusion of elements to which they object. Others simply expect consultation at a draft stage, as in the two studies reported here.

Emphasis placed on utility

An important aim throughout both studies was the importance attached by
both stakeholders and the evaluation teams to the implementation of findings
and recommendations, that is, the utility of the research. In relation to
utility, the presentation of final evaluation reports frequently has less impact
than those preceded by direct face-to-face interaction between stakeholders
and evaluators, to provide them with feedback about evaluation findings
and the nature of the data.

One important reason for involving stakeholders in face-to-face discussions of findings and recommendations is to make sure there is shared
understanding about what is meant. The purpose of this is more than a
matter of professional courtesy. The procedure acts as a way of corroborat-
ing the facts and evidence presented in the evaluation report. Comments
made by stakeholders may be helpful, not only in relation to the evaluation
analysis, but also as a way of providing feedback to the evaluation team on
the process and conduct of the evaluation. For this reason, we published
comments from stakeholders as part of final reports. Another benefit from
such consultations is that while stakeholders may still disagree with the
conclusions and interpretations of the evaluation team, they should not
disagree over the facts of the case. Perceived factual inaccuracies were raised
by stakeholders and these were settled through a search for further evidence. The opportunity to view a preliminary draft of the findings and
recommendations may also produce further evidence. In both our studies,
stakeholders remembered new relevant material that they had not reported
during the initial data gathering period.

Conclusions

Formative evaluation provides a detailed, rich description of a setting, without excluding the contextual aspects that impinge upon the lives of the
variety of stakeholding groups. At the same time, it affords the opportunity
to generate illuminative data, using systematic and triangulated approaches.
However, there is the danger that formative evaluation comes to be viewed
as a panacea for the ills of quantitative models of evaluation. The inclusion
of the context as a critical part of an evaluation creates particular challenges
and, as with other methods of inquiry, there are problems. First, difficulties
may arise at a 'paradigm level'. Evaluators may adopt different and mutu-
ally exclusive positions and reject the merits of approaches other than their

own.[31,32] This is based on the belief that the philosophies of the qualitative and quantitative research paradigms are so opposed that they cannot be mixed, and that the methods used in each are too different to use together. In common with most health care research, methods expertise in palliative care researchers has been closely tied to the methodological focus of their discipline. If evaluation in palliative care is to emerge as a truly interprofessional enterprise, a more balanced approach to methods which emphasizes methodological appropriateness will need to supplant those of conventional (and limiting) disciplinary orthodoxy.

Second, the richness and 'unpredictability' of the social context means that in this form of evaluation a great deal of data is generated. This can make data collection and analysis both difficult and time-consuming. Problems can, therefore, arise when evaluation findings must be disseminated in time for modifications to be made as a result of the evaluation. This can lead to a tension between doing something which can feed into practice quickly, and conducting a more detailed and rigorous study whose findings are out of date – and hence have little impact by the time they are reported. While it is possible to provide feedback quickly (our final report to King's Mill was delivered within four months of the study commencing) and subsequently produce a more detailed analysis (our discussion of the costs of using voluntary staff at King's Mill appeared two years later),[33] this nevertheless remains an important issue to be resolved. Great attention has to be paid, therefore, to feasibility and acceptability.

Formative evaluation relies heavily on the use of qualitative data and, in the eyes of some, there is a problem in implementing recommendations that do not rest upon the 'scientific' methods that funders, ethics committees and decision makers have come to expect. As a research endeavour, qualitative approaches have been viewed as less desirable than, for example, experiments or surveys. Two possible reasons for this include the perceived lack of rigour, and the inability of qualitative methods to provide scientific generalizations. It may prove more fruitful, however, for the relation between qualitative and quantitative methods to be characterized as complementary rather than as exclusive.[34] The two case studies described show how quantitative and qualitative work can be conducted in a complementary fashion. The complexity of the issues that surround the delivery of palliative care, coupled with the increasing acceptance of alternative methods of inquiry, means that qualitative evaluation offers particular promise and may have wider relevance for those wishing to review their service provision.

References

1 Fitzpatrick, R. and Boulton, M. (1994) Qualitative methods for assessing health care. *Quality Health Care*, 3: 107–13.

2 Clark, D. (1997) What is qualitative research and what can it contribute to palliative care? *Palliative Medicine*, 11: 159–66.

3 Ingleton, C., Field, D., Clark, D., Carradice, M. and Crowther, A. (1995) *King's Mill Hospice: Three Years On (1991–94), Occasional Paper 16*. Sheffield: Trent Palliative Care Centre.

4 Ingleton, C., White, F. and Clark, D. (1996) *What Did We Do Without It: An Evaluation of the Services Provided by Newark and District Hospice Aid (Beaumond House), Occasional Paper 18*. Sheffield: Trent Palliative Care Centre.

5 Ingleton, C., Field, D. and Clark, D. (1997) Multi-disciplinary case study as an approach to the evaluation of palliative care services: two examples. *International Journal of Palliative Nursing*, 3: 335–9.

6 Field, D., Ingleton, C. and Clark, D. (1997) The cost of unpaid labour: the use of voluntary staff in the King's Mill Hospice. *Health and Social Care in the Community*, 5: 198–208.

7 Keen, J. and Packwood, T. (1995) Case study evaluation. *British Medical Journal*, 311: 444–6.

8 Smith, G. and Cantley, C. (1991) Pluralistic evaluation, in *Evaluation: Research Highlights in Social Work 8*, 2nd edition. London: Jessica Kingsley.

9 Denzin, N.K. (1970) *The Research Act in Sociology: A Theoretical Introduction to Sociological Methods*. London: Sage.

10 Guba, E.G. and Lincoln, Y.G. (1989) *Fourth Generation Evaluation*. Beverly Hills, CA: Sage.

11 Patton, M.Q. (1980) *Qualitative Evaluation Methods*. Beverly Hills, CA: Sage.

12 Patton, M.Q. (1986) *Utilisation-focused Evaluation*. London: Sage.

13 Yin, R.K. (1994) *Case Study Research: Design and Methods*, 2nd edition. Applied social research methods series, Vol. 5. Thousand Oaks, CA: Sage.

14 Yin, R.K. (1994) *Application of Case Study Research*. Applied social research methods series, Vol. 34. Newbury Park, CA: Sage.

15 Janesick, V.J. (1994) The dance of qualitative research design: metaphor, methodolatory and meaning, in N.K. Denzin and Y.S. Lincoln (eds) *A Handbook of Qualitative Research*. London: Sage.

16 Nolan, M. and Behi, R. (1995) Triangulation: the best of both worlds? *British Journal of Nursing*, 4: 829–32.

17 Jick, T. (1979) Mixing qualitative and quantitative methods: triangulation in action. *Administrative Science Quarterly*, 24: 602–11.

18 Corner, J. (1991) In search of more complete answers to research questions: qualitative versus quantitative research methods. *Journal of Advanced Nursing*, 16: 718–27.

19 Janesick, V.J. (1994) Op. cit.

20 Campbell, D. and Fiske, D. (1959) Convergent and discriminant validation by multi-trait multi-dimensional matrix. *Psychological Bulletin*, 56: 81–105.

21 Nolan, M. and Behi, R. (1995) Op. cit.

22 Guba, E.G. and Lincoln, Y.G. (1989) Op. cit.

23 Field, D. *et al.* (1997) Op. cit.

24 Ovretveit, J. (1993) *Co-ordinating Community Care: Multidisciplinary Teams and Care Management*. Buckingham: Open University Press.

25 Hunter, S., Brace, C. and Buckley, G. (1993) The interdisciplinary assessment of older people at entry into long term institutional care: lessons from the

new community care arrangements. *Research Policy and Planning*, 11(1/2): 2–9.

26 Grayden, J.E., West, P., Galloway, S. *et al.* (1993) Bridging the gap between research and clinical practice: a collaborative approach. *Oncology Nursing Forum*, 20: 953–4.

27 Wiggington, M.A., Miracle, V.A., Sims, J. and Mitchell, K. (1994) Partners in nursing education collaborate on continuing education projects. *Journal of Nursing Staff Development*, 10: 245–7.

28 Keen, J. and Packwood, T. (1995) Op. cit.

29 Roethlisberger, F.J. and Dickson, W.J. (1947) *Management and the Worker.* Cambridge, MA: Harvard University Press.

30 James, N. (1992) A postscript to nursing, in P. Abbott and R. Sapsford (eds) *Research into Practice.* Buckingham: Open University Press.

31 Powers, B. (1987) Taking sides: a response to Goodwin and Goodwin. *Nursing Research*, 36: 122–6.

32 Goodwin, L. and Goodwin, W. (1984) Qualitative versus quantitative research or qualitative and quantitative research? *Nursing Research*, 33: 378–80.

33 Field, D. *et al.* (1997) Op. cit.

34 Pope, C. and Mays, N. (1995) Reaching the parts other methods cannot reach: an introduction to qualitative methods in health and health services research. *British Medical Journal*, 311: 42–5.

Acknowledgement

Ingleton, C., Field, D. and Clark, D. (1998) Formative evaluation and its relevance to palliative care. *Palliative Medicine*, 12: 197–203.

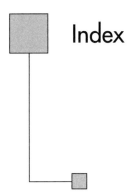

Index

Page numbers in *italics* refer to boxes and tables, *n* indicates notes.